Level Up Training Systems

Tier 1

4 Days A Week

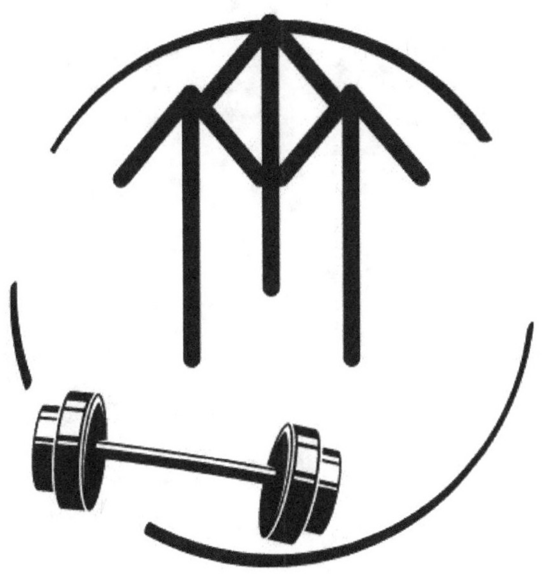

By:
JJ Jamerson

ISBN: 9798873271726

Library of Congress Control Number: 2018675309

Printed in the United States of America

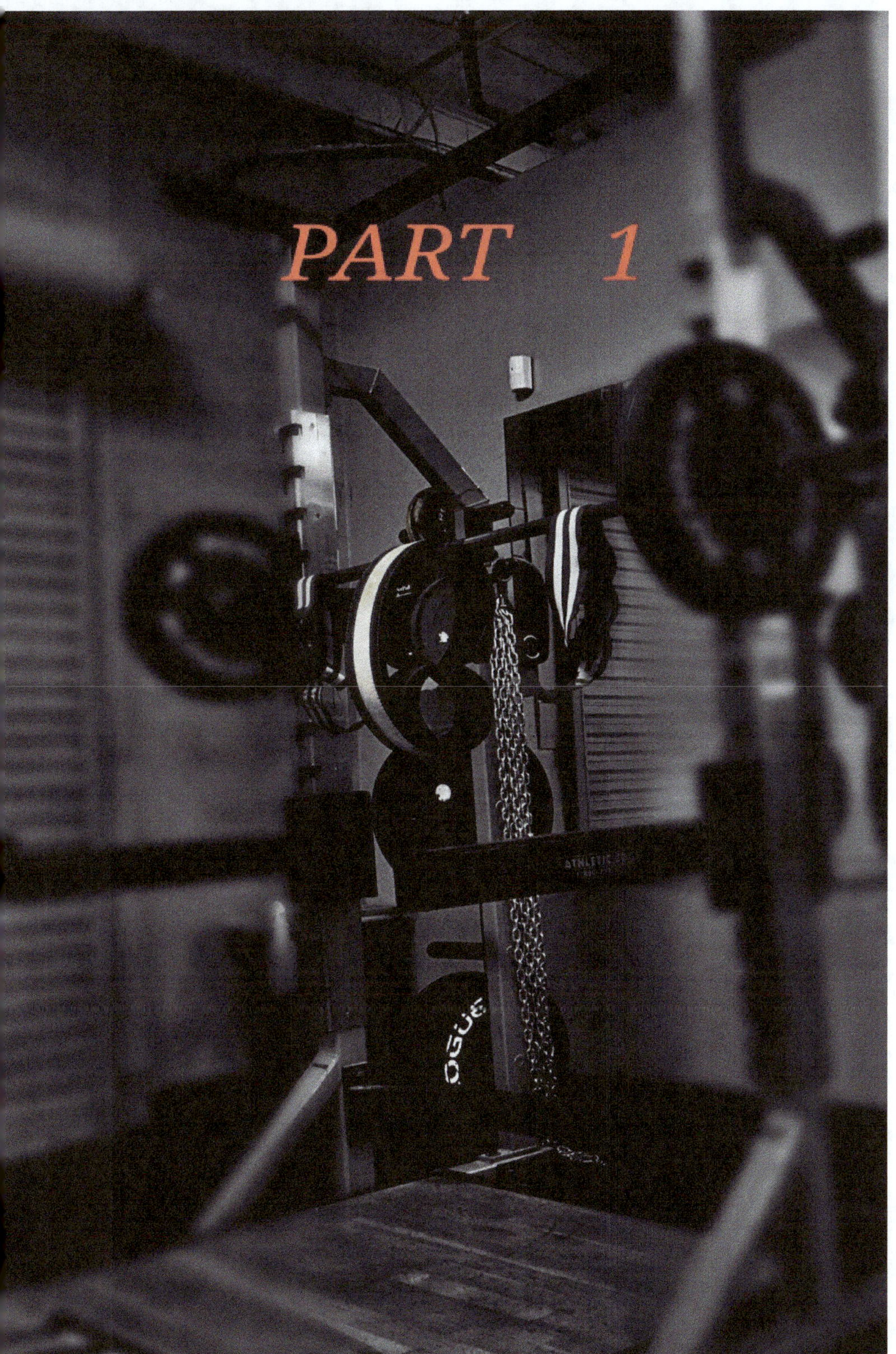
PART   1

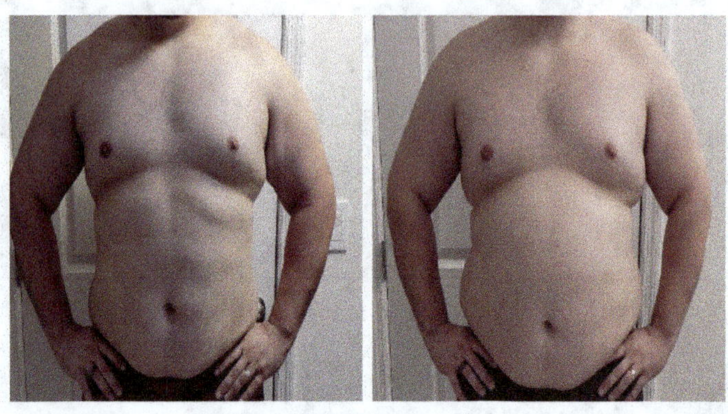

<u>Chapter 1</u>

Introduction and Disclaimer

So, you have made the decision to get back to the gym and get healthy, but you don't know where to begin? Then you have grabbed the right book! If you are anything like me, you have been here before. You have gone through the cycles. You decide to go back to the gym to get healthy, lose weight, or even get stronger. You begin going, but you do not know what to do so you wing it. You have been doing well for about a month or two but are not really seeing results.

One day, you decide to skip a day. I mean what is one day, right? That one day becomes two, then before you know it, a week has passed. Suddenly you have a gym membership you never use. I have been here before, so I know the feeling. The key to breaking this cycle was finding a style of training that I enjoy as well as a good, structured program to follow. My goal with this book is to help you with some general and simplified knowledge and a structured program that you can easily follow.

I do recommend reading the information provided. It can help you with the program and help you achieve your goals. If you would like to go straight to the program and begin your training, you can find the complete program in the back of the book. I recognize that there is a lot of information, and it can be overwhelming so, I tried to simplify the information as much as possible to make it easier to understand.

As always see a medical care provider before beginning any type of physical activity. The exercises in this book and programming are done at your discretion. When participating in any exercise or training there is a risk of physical injury. Understand you do so at your own risk. The information presented is meant to help guide you through practices that can help you achieve your goals through proper use. The information, however, does not promise any benefits when misused or misinterpreted.

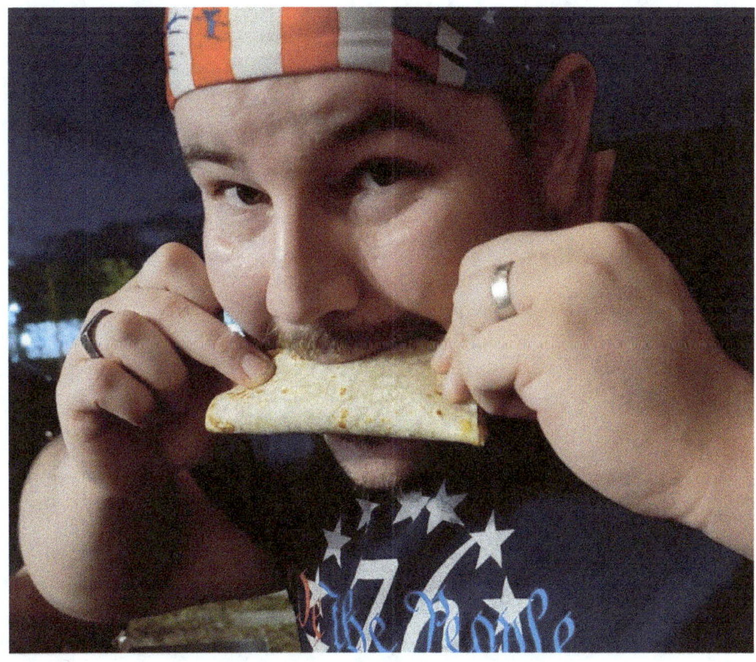

Chapter 2
General Nutrition – Bulkin or Cutting

Ah yes, the best part of the entire process! What to eat to achieve your goals. Despite the numerous diets, fads, and opinions on this topic, it really is quite simple. Multiple medical studies have proven repeatedly, calories in vs calories out is the key to weight loss/weight gain. You must burn more calories than you eat to lose weight and you must eat more calories than you burn to gain weight.

How do we calculate how many calories to eat to achieve our goals? There are apps that can do this for you such as MyFitnessPal. A nutritionist or a dietician could also give you this data. A simpler, but not as accurate way, is to take your weight and multiply it by 12.5.

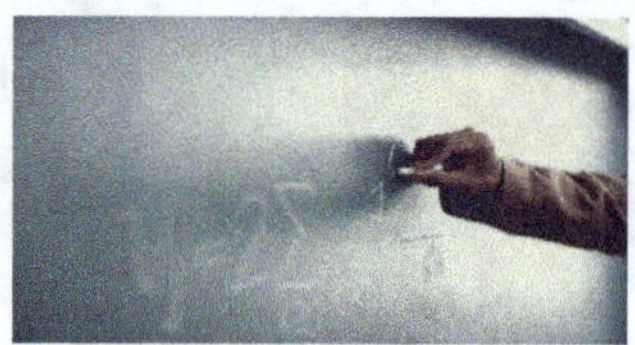

Example: Someone weights 205lbs. 205x12.5= 2,562

This means that a person weighing 205lbs could eat 2,562 calories a day and maintain their current weight. To lose weight, we would simply subtract 300-500 calories from that original number. At 205lbs with no exercise and eating 2,200 calories a day, a person should lose roughly 1-2lbs a week (Give or take some calories and pounds)

See! Super simple right? Keep in mind the formula must be updated as you lose weight, and the calories must keep going down until you meet your goal.

Example: Let's say after 8 weeks the 205lbs person has lost 20lbs. Well, 185x12.5=2,312.

Now the person who lost weight is only in a 100-calorie deficit if they stay at the same calorie intake. To continue losing weight they would need to drop down to 2,000 calories per day. This is all without exercise. In general, an average person burns anywhere from 200 to 400 calories in one hour of exercise. How many calories you burn depends on intensity and type of training. Let's say you go to the gym 4 days a week and burn 300 calories each time. Now you have increased your deficit on those days.

Example: 2,000 calories eaten is a 300-calorie deficit for a 185lbs person. They perform 1 hour of exercise burning 300 calories. They are now at 1,700 calories that day, and a 600-calorie deficit.

I understand this is a lot of information. But it is quite simple, especially with apps to track food and exercise for you.

This is where this gets a little more complicated but that's ok because I am going to give you the formula to make it work so you can still enjoy some pizza and beer on the weekend!

The solution to this is that you need to think of a calorie deficit more on a weekly scale than a daily scale. We will keep with the same 205lbs person. They need to eat 2,200 calories a day to lose weight. Weekly they need to consume 15,400 calories to be in a calorie deficit of 2,500 calories for the week, or 350 calorie deficits daily. I know this seems more confusing, but it makes it easier to plan. Let's say you cut an extra 200 calories out each day Mon-Fri. This would give you an extra 1,000 calories to use on Saturday or Sunday.

<u>Example</u>: Full Week eating!

Monday	Tuesday	Wednesday	Thursday	Friday	Saturday	Sunday
2,000	2,000	2,000	2,000	2,000	2,900	2,500

15,400 calorie weeks. 2,500 calorie deficits.

Monday	Tuesday	Wednesday	Thursday	Friday	Saturday	Sunday
2,200	2,200	2,200	2,200	2,200	2,200	2,200

Still at 15,400 calories. Still in a 2,500-calorie deficit for the week. Now you get to enjoy that pizza and beer on Saturday. You still must stay within those calorie goals for Saturday and Sunday, but this allows you to have foods you enjoy.

This method can be used any way you want. Eat less on Monday because you know you're going to Disney's Food and Wine Festival the next day. So on and so on. Any combination works if the weekly deficit is met.

<u>Note:</u> Same rules apply to bulking. If you're underweight or a skinny kid trying to beef up, just reverse the process. Instead of subtracting 300-500 calories, add them. Still take your weight and multiply by 12.5. Then eat and eat some more.

By this point you're probably thinking to yourself, "I thought he was just going to tell me what to eat, not make me do math." Unfortunately, I cannot do that as it requires certain certifications and a degree in nutrition. I am only certified in training, but I can share general advice.

Pro Tip: A grilled chicken sandwich with a 12-count grilled nugget on the side with a side salad and a diet coke is only 600 calories and 70 grams of protein. Use the buffalo sauce on the grilled meat for added flavor and no added calories.

Macros, otherwise known as macronutrients, are proteins, carbohydrates, and fats. These are found in all foods. Your body uses each of these nutrients differently.

- Proteins are used in muscle synthesis. They help rebuild muscles that are damaged. When performing exercises and resistance training, this is the most important macro to track. Recommended 1.2-1.4 grams of protein per pound of body weight. 1 gram of protein = 4 calories. So, 100 grams of protein equals 400 calories.

- Carbohydrates are used for energy. This is the body's primary source of energy. These are what are going to get you through those workouts. Carbs do tend to make the body retain water, which is why it is important to hydrate when doing keto. It is also why some people lose so much weight on keto. Most of that is water weight. Carbs can also make you feel bloated. 1 gram of Carbs = 4 calories. So, 100 grams of carbs equals 400 calories.

- Fats are used as a source of energy and to protect organs. They also help your body absorb nutrients and produce hormones. 1 gram of fat = 9 calories. So, 100 grams of fats equals 900 calories.

There are several diets that use strategies that include keeping one or another of these macronutrients low. Low fat diets for the longest time were the most widely used, but diets like Keto have become very popular in recent years. These diets work by keeping low or outright excluding fats and carbs. By doing this they put the body in a calorie deficit because you are no longer getting calories from the macro. This is why low-fat diets work so well. By keeping fats low, it allows you to eat more without going over your calorie goals.

Regardless of what diet you use, the goal of remaining in a calorie deficit is still the most important thing. Proteins should always be prioritized as well, especially if you are performing resistance training. As always, do your research and speak to your healthcare provider before changing your diet. Depending on your health, certain diets might not be good for you.

Below I will give a few examples of a week of eating for a person cutting. We will continue to use the 205lbs person as an example.

Example:

Low Fat Diet –

Macro	Monday	Tuesday	Wednesday	Thursday	Friday	Saturday	Sunday
Grams	2,200	2,200	2,200	2,200	2,200	2,200	2,200
Proteins	245g	250g	220g	240g	260g	250g	200g
Carbs	200g	180g	180g	205g	200g	150g	230g
Fats	45g	56g	69g	45g	25g	66g	50g

Keto Diet –

Macro	Monday	Tuesday	Wednesday	Thursday	Friday	Saturday	Sunday
Grams	2,200	2,200	2,200	2,200	2,200	2,200	2,200
Proteins	250g	250g	250g	250g	250g	250g	250g
Carbs	5g	5g	5g	5g	5g	5g	5g
Fats	130g	130g	130g	130g	130g	130g	130g

Normal Mixed Diet –

Macro	Monday	Tuesday	Wednesday	Thursday	Friday	Saturday	Sunday
Grams	2,200	2,200	2,200	2,200	2,200	2,200	2,200
Proteins	250g	250g	250g	250g	250g	250g	250g
Carbs	150g	120g	100g	100g	120g	150g	90g
Fats	66g	80g	88g	88g	80g	66g	93g

Extra – Carb Loading diet -

Macro	Monday	Tuesday	Wednesday	Thursday	Friday	Saturday	Sunday
Grams	2,200	2,200	2,200	2,200	2,200	2,200	2,200
Proteins	250g	250g	250g	250g	250g	250g	250g
Carbs	5g	5g	250g	5g	5g	250g	5g
Fats	130g	130g	25g	130g	130g	25g	130g

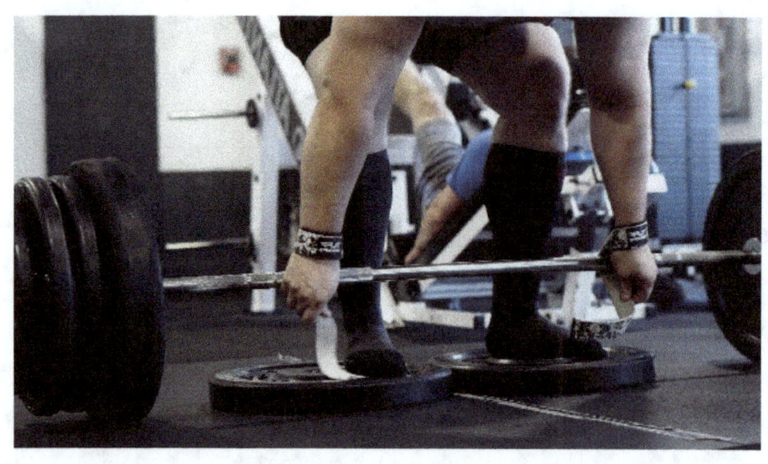

Chapter 3
General Lifting Advice

We are finally done with the fun stuff, now on to the lifting. Oh! You didn't think nutrition was fun? I always have fun talking about food!

Doubtlessly you have heard different advice or opinions regarding exercise and fitness. There is so much information from so many diverse sources, it can be hard to know what is right and what is wrong. I am going to do my best to give you general advice to help you on your journey. The advice I give is based on my own experience, and on scientific data that I have studied and learned through multiple sources.

We will start with the simplest advice first. What to wear and gear you will need for lifting:

- Clothing: You can wear whatever you are most comfortable in. Shorts and a t-shirt, Leggings and a sports bra, or sweats and an oversized shirt. Whatever you are most comfortable wearing, although it should be something flexible and made for active movements. So, while there are no rules for working out in jeans it should probably be avoided.

- Shoes: In general, you will want a flat soled shoe for lifting. These can be vans or special shoes. Just search deadlift shoes online and find a pair you like. These shoes are great for all lifting. After lifting for a while you may notice you have trouble squatting to depth. A good pair of squat shoes with a raised heel can help with this but aren't necessary.

- Socks: Whatever you want. Although if you are doing deadlifts, you may want a knee-high sock or a deadlift sock. You can avoid this though, by just wearing pants or leggings.

- Gloves: This is the controversial one. I say do what makes you happy. Some people will argue that you shouldn't wear gloves when lifting. "It's more '*MaNlY*' without gloves. You must build those calluses." But not everyone wants ripped up callused hands. So do what you feel comfortable doing and ignore them.

- Lifting Belt: These are not necessary but are a great tool. I recommend waiting to get one until you have built a solid foundation first. A belt simply allows you to brace your core more effectively. It increases the inter abdominal pressure to tense the muscle in the core to support proper posture during lifts. If you do get one, go with a prong or lever belt. Velcro belts are not as good at getting tight and helping you brace.

- Knee sleeves/braces: If you have knee pain or discomfort, see a medical professional. With that said, for legal reasons, sleeves and braces are great. They give compression on the joints and support for the lift. There are a lot of different types out there, but neoprene knee sleeves are the best, in my opinion.

- Bands: Most gyms will have these somewhere for use. You can get your own set if you want to be extra like I am. These are one of my favorite tools to use. They are very versatile and especially great for warmups. I use bands in the program, but I also offer alternatives.

- Deadlift Straps: There are pros and cons to these. On the one hand they help with grip while performing some exercise. On the other hand, they limit your grip strength growth. You're only as strong as your weakest link but at the same time why should you limit growth of larger muscle because of smaller muscles. At the end of the day this is one that comes down to your discretion.

Overall, do what makes you happy and wear whatever you're comfortable in. Use whatever gear you like that makes the lift easier, or more comfortable. If at any time while lifting you feel a sharp pain, you should stop immediately. Discomfort and general aches and soreness are to be expected from exercises. You should push through that, however, if you feel actual pain, then you should stop immediately and seek medical advice.

Another helpful thing you can do is to record your lifts. Specifically, from the side angle. Not to post, unless you want to, but to see your own lifts. Without a coach there to observe you and correct technique and form, you must be your own coach. The only way to know exactly how the lift looks is to be able to go back and see yourself performing it. This may be a controversial topic in the gym, but it is a great tool to use.

When it comes to technique and form, things get a bit more complicated. Everyone's body is different, which changes how lifts will look. Length of femur in proportion to torso changes how squats and deadlifts look. How the femur attaches to the hip can change whether you should use a close stance or wider stance with squats. I know you're not here for a full anatomy lesson so I will keep it simple with the breakdown of each lift. Do what feels most comfortable and allows you to perform the lift through a full range of motion.

During all your lifts, you should be focused on the feel of the muscle and on your breathing. During big compound lifts you should be bracing your core. This requires breathing into your abdomen and flexing all the muscles of your core. Bracing your core is what you do if someone were to hit you in the belly or if you bear down. What you're doing is tightening not only your abdominal muscles but the muscles that surround your spine. The combination of the full lungs and the braced core provides the maximum rigidity for your torso.

In the program, I will use squats, bench, and deadlifts. Below I will show you variations of each that you can use at your discretion. You may feel more comfortable performing one variation over another. Have fun and experiment with each to find what you like. I will also give pros and cons for each and how they change the stimulus to the muscles.

The Squat:

My least favorite of the big 3. Coincidently, it is also the one I am best at. A lot of people complain about bad knees or knee pain from squatting. This is typically due to bad technique or other factors. The squat itself is a great exercise and if done right can make your knees stronger. There are 2 major variations of the squat: high bar and Low bar squats. The choice is yours on which you want to use. Whatever you choose, stick with that variation through the full 20 weeks before switching. The difference between the two is the placement of the bar on the back as well as an emphasis on muscles used. The squat is primarily a quad movement; however, it does use the hamstrings and glutes as well. Changing bar placement and technique can change how much other muscles are used.

When high bar squatting, the bar rests on top of your traps. This is the most common style that you see. The position of the bar allows you to stand more upright and puts more emphasis on the quads. The low bar squat has the bar resting lower on the back. The bar should rest right below the traps and on top of the rear delts. This will change the center of gravity for the squat. You will lean over more, and it will put more emphasis on the hips. Hand placement should be right outside of shoulders; however, you can go wider if this is uncomfortable on your shoulders and arms. Play with hand width to find what works for you. Typically, you can squat more weight in a low bar style, but it does require a little more technique.

See Pictures for reference below:

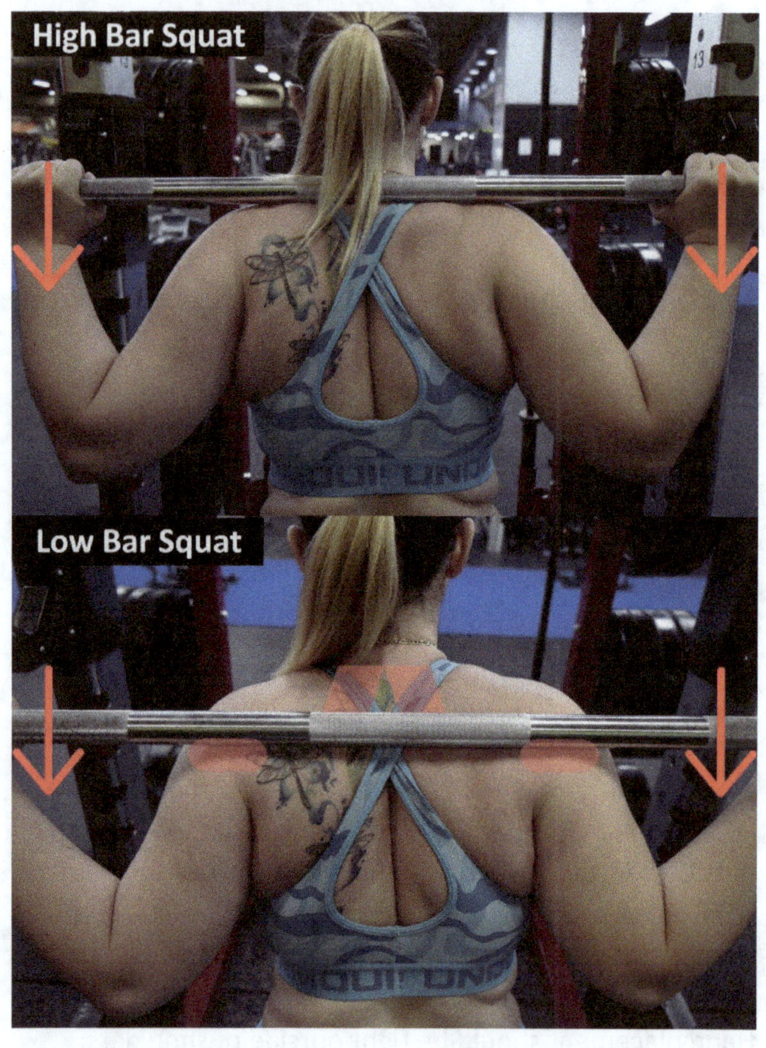

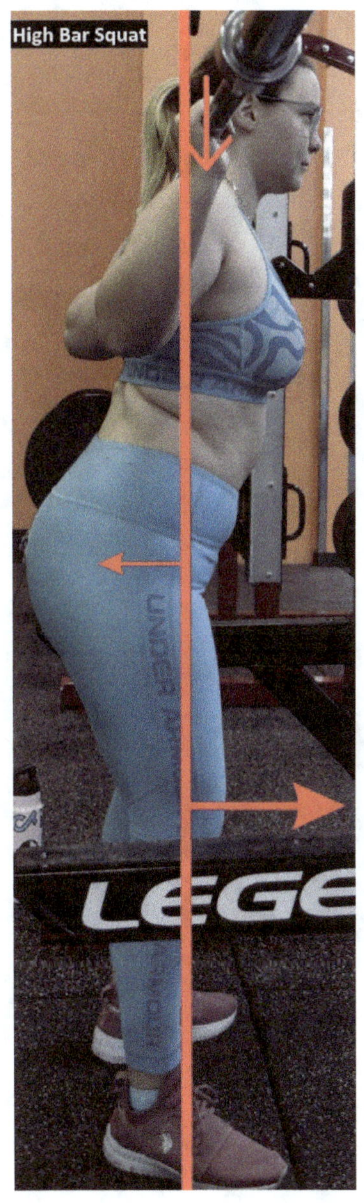

High Bar Squat

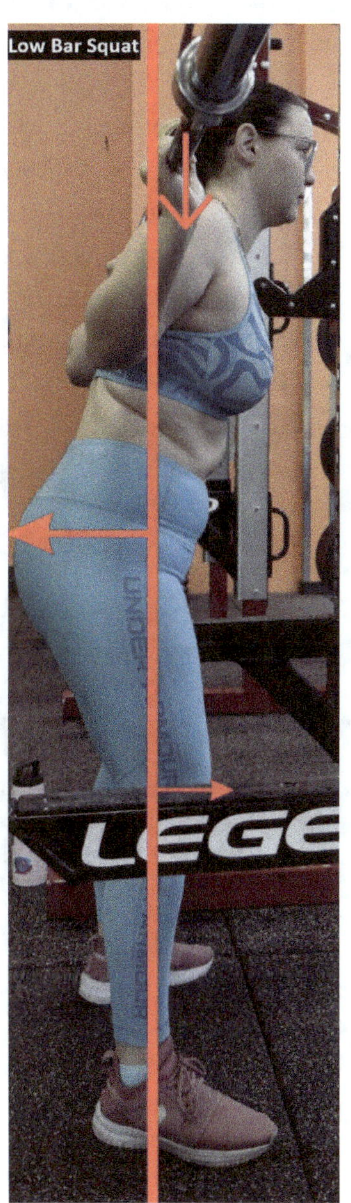

Low Bar Squat

The last type of squat that can be used requires a special bar that a lot of gyms do not have. I will include it as an option, and you can try it out if your gym happens to have one. This type of squat is an SSB Squat (squat safety bar). The bar has pads and arms that go to the front of you allowing the bar to sit on your shoulders without needing your arms pulled back. This is great for people who have bad shoulder mobility. The weight also sits more forward. This means when you squat down, the weight will pull you forward putting more emphasis on the hips and erectors. *See Pictures below for reference:*

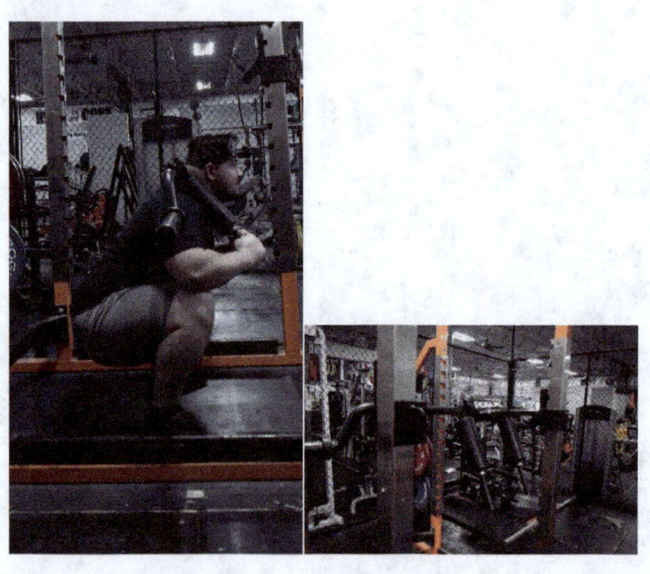

	Pros	Cons	Muscle Emphasis
High Bar	Easier to perform. Most common (meaning a higher likelihood of person having performed before.)	Generally, cannot lift as much. Uncomfortable on traps. Requires more ankle mobility for knees to go over toes.	Quads
Low Bar	Can generally move more weight.	Requires more technical know-how. Can be awkward at first due to starting more bent over. Puts more strain on shoulders and arms.	Hamstrings, Glutes
SSB Squat	Easiest to learn due to not requiring hand placement. Can still be performed even with and injured arm or shoulder.	Bars are not common in most gyms. Due to weight being more forward can put more strain on lower back.	Quads, Erectors

The next important thing is feet placement. How far apart should your feet be? This will depend on your individual hip anatomy. I recommend staring with your feet at shoulder width. Perform a squat without the bar and, once you get to a certain depth, if you feel a tightness in your hip then try a slightly wider stance. Play with feet placement until you find what is comfortable but allows full range of motion.

The last thing we will go over is the actual movement. When you un-rack the bar you should only take one step out followed by the other foot. Do not walk 5 steps back so that you are completely out of the rack. Remember, you must walk all that way back to re-rack the weight. Once you have walked the squat out, you will adjust your feet placement. Screw your feet into the ground like you are trying to turn your feet out. They should not move, but you should feel the muscles in your hips tighten and your knees rotate. Pull the bar into your back squeezing your back muscles, then push your hips back and bend your knees. Squat as deep as you are comfortable going while maintaining a tight back and pushing your knees out. When you go to stand up, imagine pushing your chest up to the ceiling.

The Bench Press:

Ah yes, the bench press. The lift all the "Bro's" use to determine strength. Honestly, when it comes to upper body strength and development, the bench press is undefeated. Some may argue that an overhead press is more functional, as you are more likely to pick something up and place it above your head than you are to push something heavy away from you. However, the bench press is still an amazingly useful tool, whether for strength gains or general fitness.

There are many people who avoid the bench press. Some do not use it due to shoulder issues, while others do not think it has many benefits. With proper technique and load management, the lift is safe for the shoulder joint and there are many benefits to the bench press.

When performing the bench press, lay down with your back on the bench. Grab the bar with a full grip and thumbs around the bar. Pull back and squeeze your shoulder blades together to create tension. Using your legs, drive your heels into the ground and push back into your traps. Make sure your butt is on the bench. Straighten your arms and un-rack the bar, bringing it over your chest. While maintaining tension in your back and legs, lower the bar to your chest. Attempt to bend the bar with your hands and tuck your elbow in roughly at a 45-degree angle to your body and bring the bar all the way to your chest. Your arms should be parallel with each other at the bottom of the lift. Pause slightly, then in one fluid motion, squeeze your glutes, drive your heels into to the ground and yeet the bar off your chest.

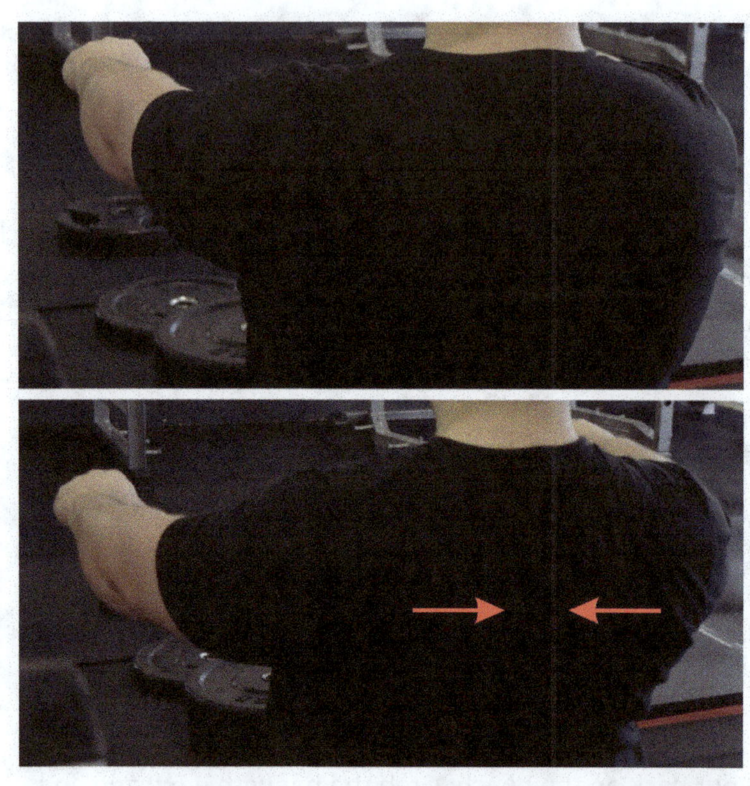

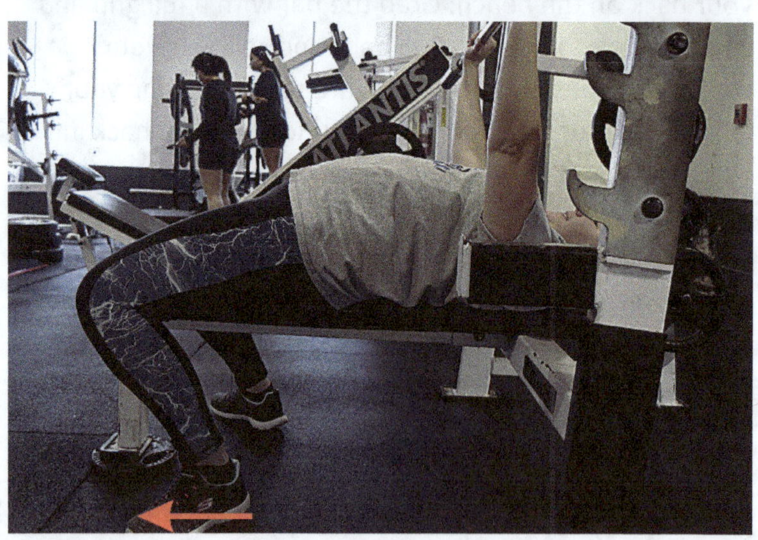

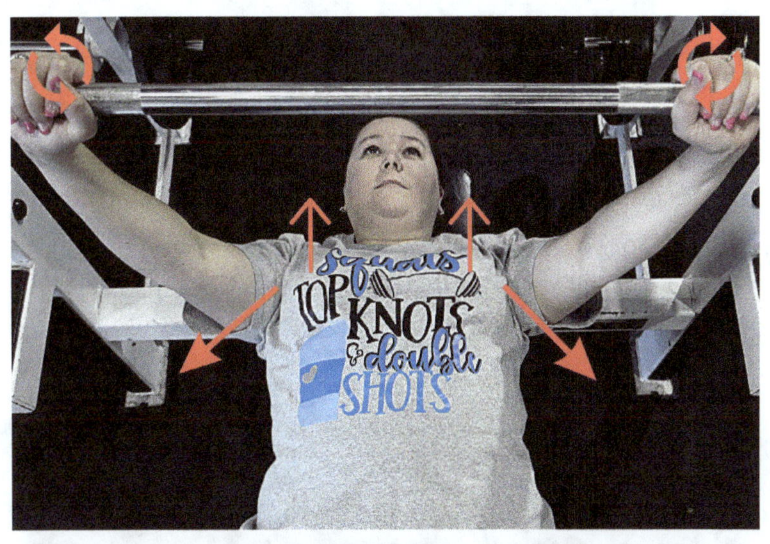

squats
TOP KNOTS
& double
SHOTS

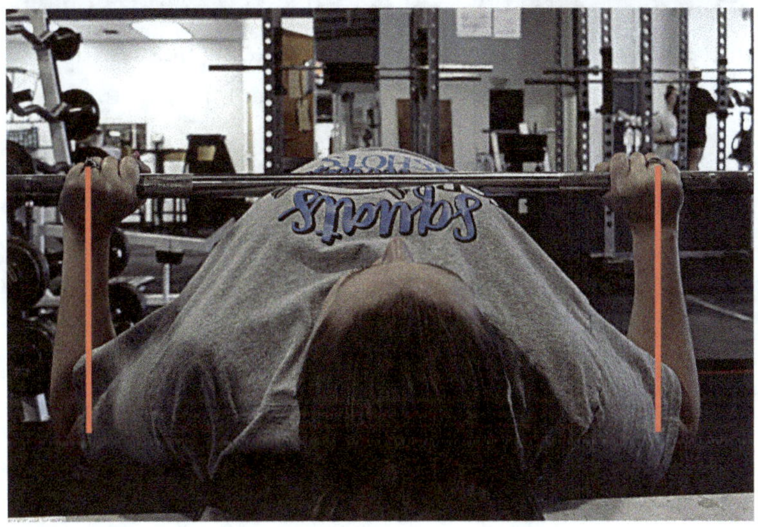

The Deadlift:

Arguably one of the best lifts for everything is the deadlift. From a functional standpoint, you often need to bend over to pick something up. From a strength standpoint, it uses your entire body to move lots of weight. From a weight loss standpoint, it uses lots of muscles to burn tons of calories. Whatever your goal is, deadlifts can help.

Deadlifts have a bit of a reputation as an injury prone exercise. However, if done correctly with good technique and without trying to go too heavy, then they are perfectly safe. This applies to almost everything you do in the gym. Proper technique and not going heavier than you are prepared for is key to remaining injury free.

There are three main deadlift variations. These variations are Conventional, Sumo, and trap bar deadlifts. It is up to you to decide which you want to use. Whatever your choice, stick with that technique through the entire program. The variation of deadlifts, like squats, do change the main muscles used so it is important to stick with the same one throughout.

<u>Conventional Deadlifts:</u>

When setting up a conventional deadlift, you want your feet to be roughly shoulder width apart. The bar should be over the middle of your foot or roughly an inch from your shin. You should then bend over and grab the bar. Extend your thumbs where the tip of your thumb is in the middle of your shin and wrap your thumb around the bar. Your shins should still be about an inch from the bar. Pull the slack out of the bar while pulling your shoulders down and back. You should hear a slight cling from the bar and the weights. Lower your hips down until you feel your shins touch the bar then imagine pushing your hips forward and pushing the floor away. Your hands should be attempting to bend the bar around your shins and should maintain contact with your shins/legs all the way up. Set the bar down the same way while maintaining contact with your legs. This can be a bit uncomfortable as the bar is basically dragging up and down your legs, which is why deadlift socks, leggings, or pants are recommended.

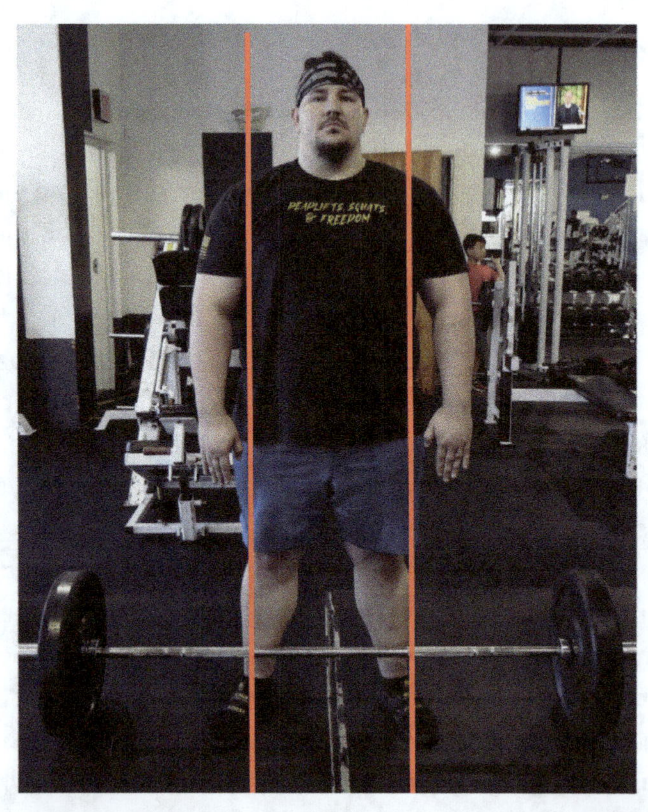

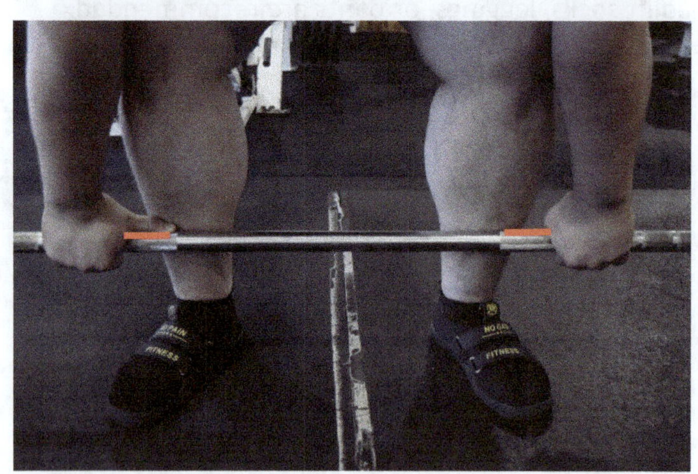

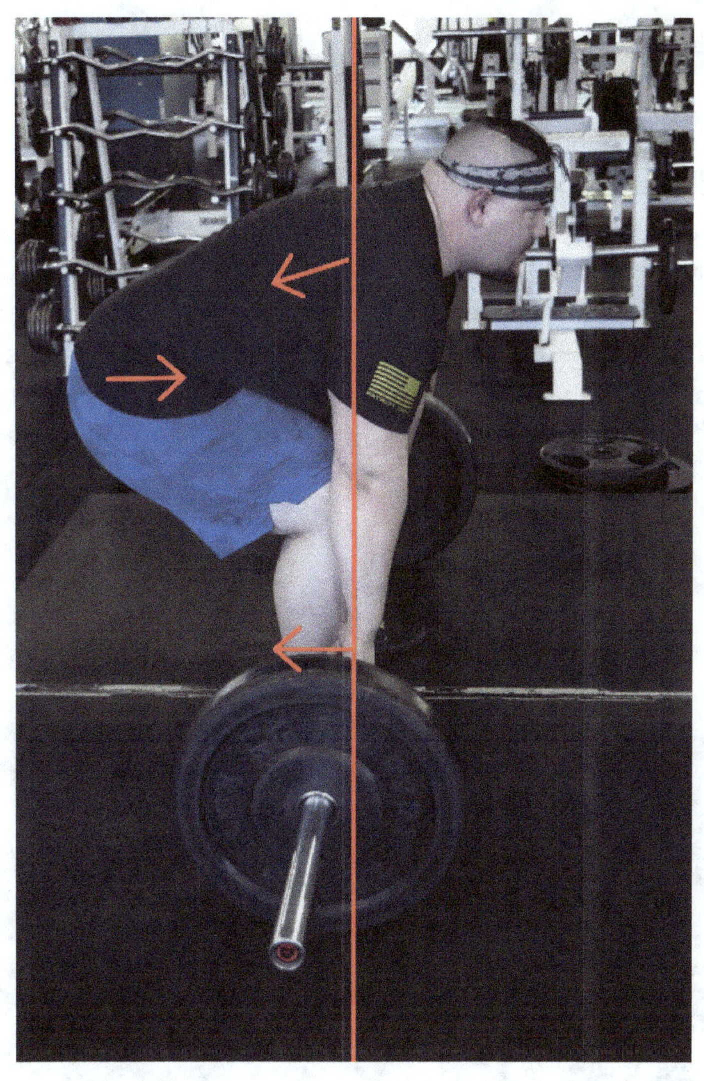

Sumo Deadlifts:

Sumo deadlifts are like conventional deadlifts in execution; however, your feet are wider and pushing out. Your feet should be pointing outward, and your shins should be parallel with each other. You then want to let your arms hang naturally down and squat down to the bar while keeping your torso as upright as possible. Grab the bar and use it to pull yourself down while also pulling the slack from the bar. Now that you are in position, you want to squeeze your glutes and push your hips through.

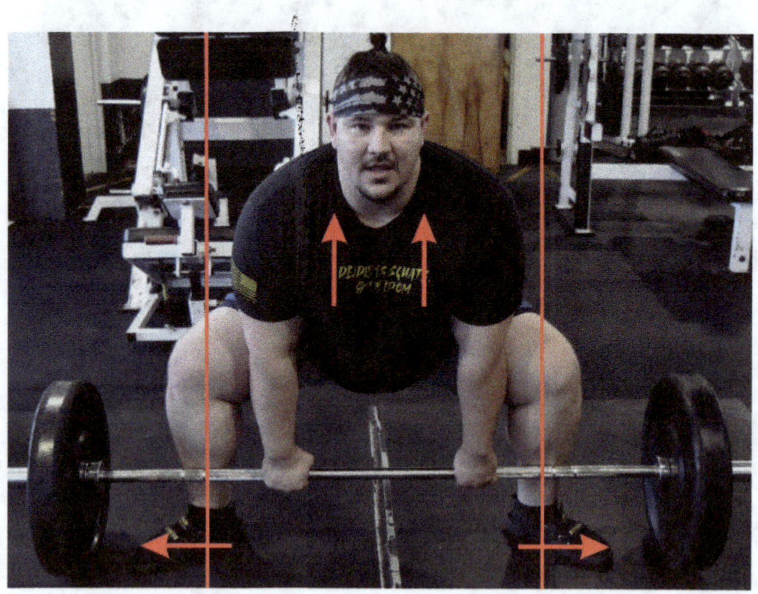

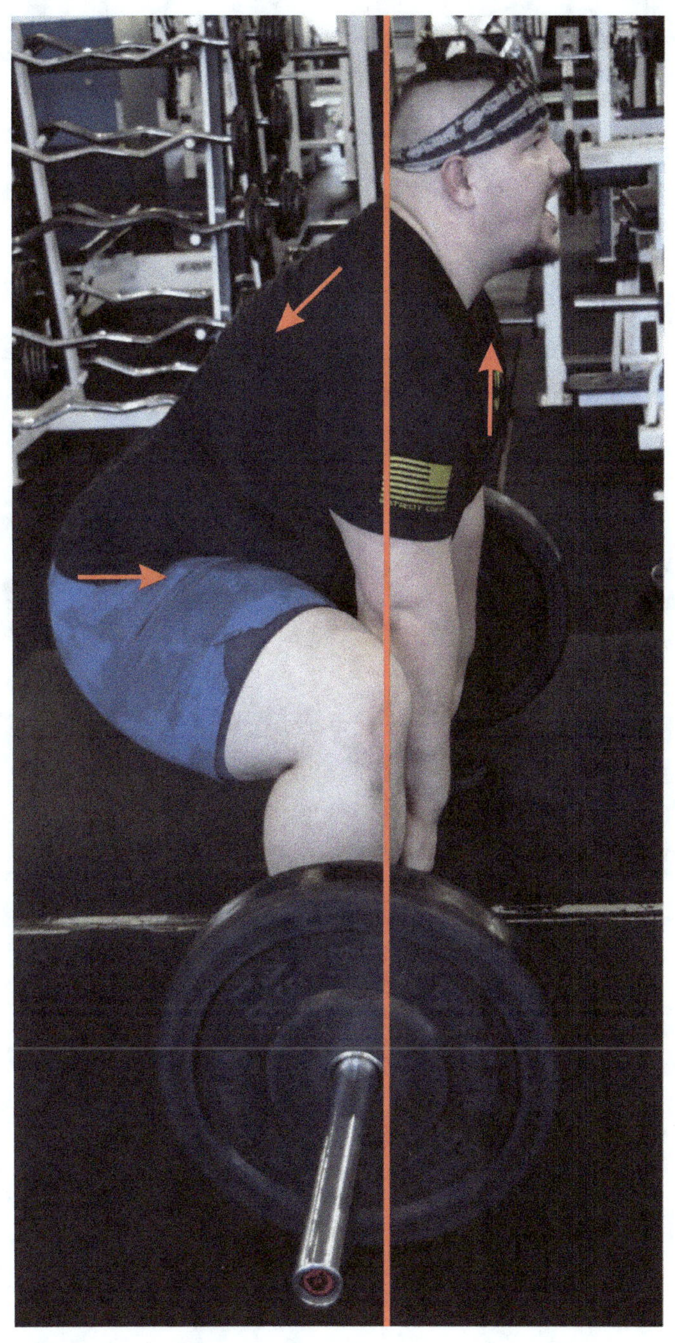

<u>Trap Bar Deadlifts:</u>

The trap bar is the last variation and is considered the safest and easiest to learn. To begin you should step into the trap bar. You should stand directly in the middle of bar with the weights at center foot. Stand tall and straight with your hands directly by your side. Squat down and grab the handles. Squeeze your glutes and push your hips forward while keeping your chest high.

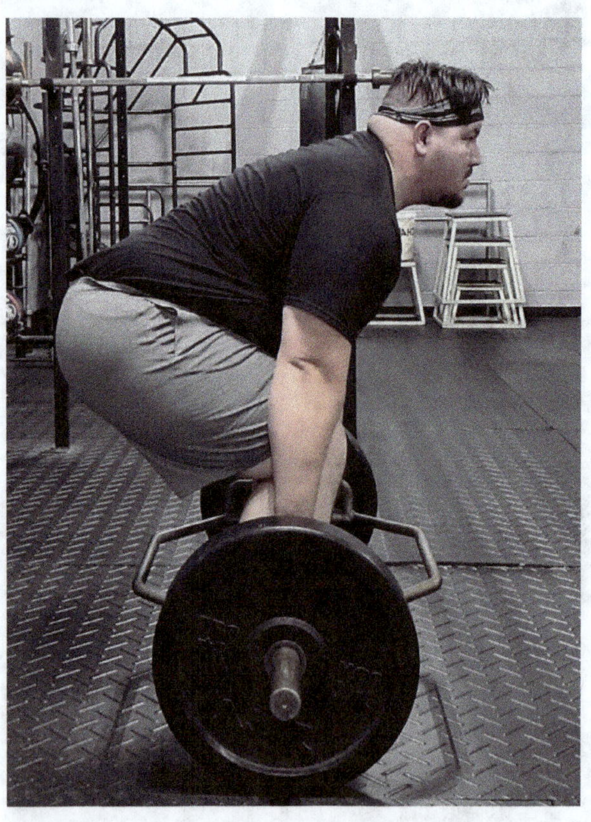

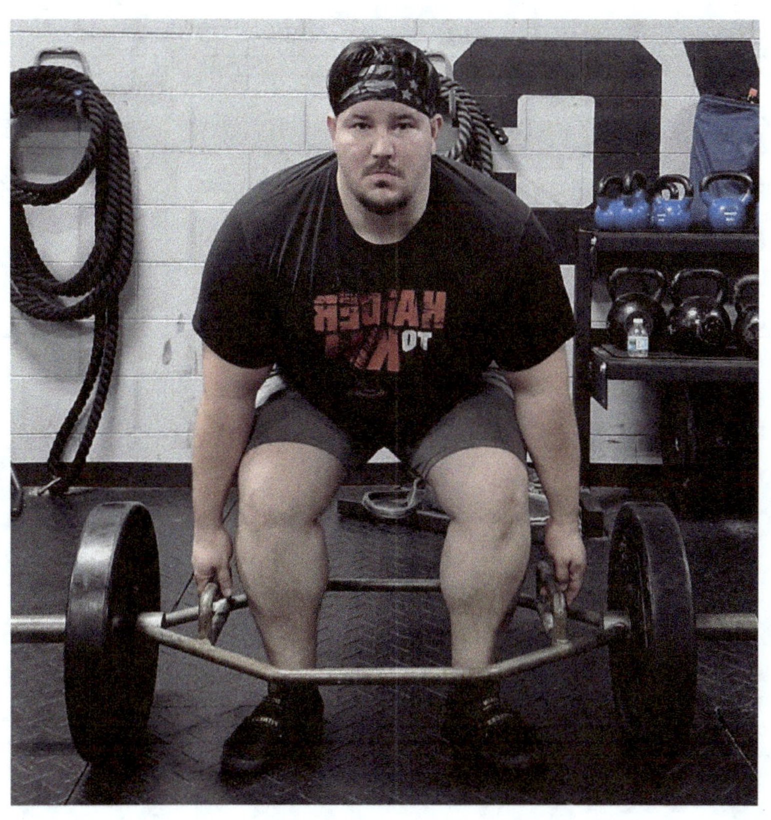

	Pros	Cons	Muscle Emphasis
Conventional	Standard and most functional. Great for building a strong back.	Technical	Glutes, Erectors, hamstrings
Sumo	More focus on legs and hips and less strain on lower back(erectors) Can generally move more weight.	Harder to learn and get "right." Most technical of the 3	Glutes, Quads, Adductors
Trap Bar	"Safest." Easiest to learn. Less strain on erectors	Does not give same stimulus nor as functional as other variations.	Glutes, Quads

Mastering these three lifts will translate to nearly every other lift you do inside the gym. Whether you are dumbbell benching or doing squats on a machine. The same general principles apply. Maintaining a good brace, and general tightness in your core is necessary for all lifts.

Mentality:

The last thing I want to go over is mentality. I know what you're thinking, "oh God, self-help." Just think, you get a fitness book and a self-help book for the price of one. That's a win! I won't go on a whole self-help tangent, but I will try to give you some advice that has helped me stay active in fitness.

The biggest tip I can give is to prioritize the gym. Pick a time you want to go and do everything in your power to get there. There will be days you're not going to want to go and that is ok. Just tell yourself you will go to the parking lot and sit, then maybe get some Chick-fil-a for comfort. Most of the time once you are at the parking lot you will just go in and workout. Then you can get some Chick-fil-a afterwards as a reward for going.

Pro Tip: A grilled chicken sandwich with a 12-count grilled nugget on the side with a side salad and a diet coke is only 600 calories and 70 grams of protein. Use the buffalo sauce on the grilled meat for added flavor and no added calories.

It is ok to half-butt a workout. I know I am speaking blasphemy, but it needs to be said. If you are having an off day and just do not have the necessary energy to put everything into a workout, that is ok. A crappy workout is better than no workout.

Learn to enjoy the process. It may suck during the workout but, the high you feel after makes it worth it. The sense of accomplishment, of having done something hard you did not want to do, can give you a huge boost. This is especially useful when dealing with mental health. Studies have shown that exercise can help with many mental health issues, such as depression, anxiety, and bi-polar disorder. I could break down the science behind it but instead I will speak from personal experience.

I spoke about the feeling of accomplishment giving you a high after. This has helped me break through depression. I have often had that feeling of wanting to do something but, just not having the energy to get up and do it. Lifting weights has helped me break through that mindset. I had to force myself up and get to the parking lot. That is the start.

I also understand the high anxiety. The constant battle with your own brain is exhausting. I can channel and take all those negative emotions out on the weights. The weights won't break when I slam them. By the time I finish and leave the gym, all I feel is numb and my brain is quiet.

The gym is my me time. It's my time to focus on myself. This is just another way to view the gym rather than as a task to be completed.

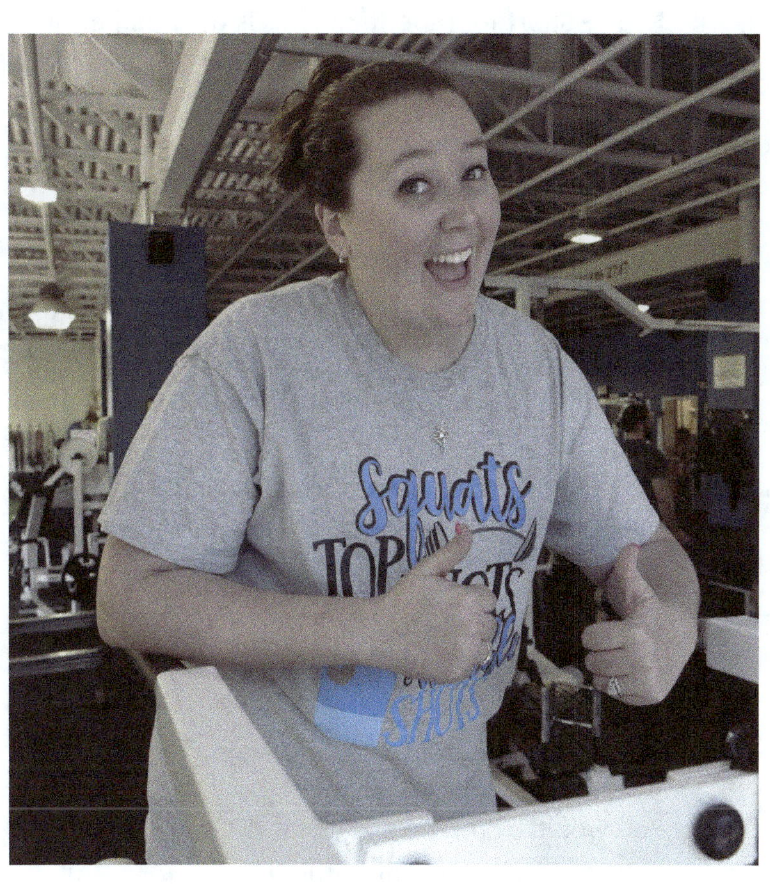

Squats
TOP
SHO

Chapter 4

Explanation of Program Format

<u>Explanation of Terms:</u>

- Reps – Short for repetition. This is the number of times in a single go that you will perform an exercise. This means if the program says do 10 pushups. 10 would be the number of repetitions you would perform.
- Sets – This is the number of times you will perform the exercise for the set amount of Reps. This means that if the program says to perform pushups for 2 sets of 10 reps. You would perform 10 pushups, rest, then perform 10 more pushups and be done.
- DB or BB – This is short for Dumbbell (DB) or Barbell (BB). This shows what you should use in the given exercise.
- AMAP – short for as many as possible. This indicates that you should perform as many reps as possible until you cannot perform another rep.
- Tempo – This indicates the speed of the rep. Say the program calls for a 5,3,0 tempo on pushups. You would begin the pushup at the top. Lower yourself with a 5 count to the bottom, pause for 3 counts, then pushup as fast as possible.

<u>**Program Format:**</u>

The program is set up as a 4-day split. This means there are 4 days that you will need to go to the gym to get the full benefits. Each day has a specific focus:

1.   Bench, Chest, and Arms
2.   Squats, Quads, and Back
3.   Shoulders and Arms
4.   Deadlifts and Back

Some of the exercises in the program will say banded. If your gym does not have bands, it is perfectly acceptable to use a cable machine as an alternative.

By the end of the week, you will have hit every muscle group multiple times. What days you want to go are completely up to you. I personally like going Mon, Tues, Thurs, and Fri. What time you go is also up to you. Before work or after work, early morning or late in the evening. Each block of training will last four weeks. Three weeks followed by a one-week deload. I will go over the deload week in more detail later in the book.

You may notice in the program that reps show two numbers. This is referred to as a rep range. The goal with this is to strive for the larger number. You will increase the weight each set and attempt to hit the higher number. If you miss the higher number, it is fine as long as you do not go lower than the small number. Once you have failed to hit the higher number, you do not increase the weight any further. You will complete your remaining sets at that weight.

Example:

The program has the DB bench press for 5x10-12 for you to complete that day. Your first set you complete 20lbs for 12 reps. Your next set you complete 25lbs for 12 reps. On your 3rd set you only manage 11 reps with 30lbs. You will now stay at 30lbs for your remaining 2 sets.

If you perform a set and go lower than the small number, you will then decrease the weight back 1 set.

Example:

On the 4th set with 30lbs you only complete 9 reps. For your 5th and last set, you will drop back to 25lbs and attempt to hit the high number again.

Every day will begin with mobility and activation. This is also known as the warm-up. The goal is to get your body loose and ready to work. Typically, you will perform three exercises designed to work on your mobility, and to get you primed and warmed up to perform.

Example:

Mobility and Activation		
IYT Raises Chest Supported	2	6-8
Dislocations	2	6-8
Pushups	2	8-12

Feel free to do more mobility work if you think you need to. I will include some mobility exercises in Appendix A. The core and activation are important to perform, as it helps to build your mobility and allows you to move without pain or discomfort. It will also help you to build up your joint strength as well as fix imbalances. This part should take only 10-15 minutes to perform.

The next part of the program is the resistance training. This is the main workout of the day. Each day has a focus as I said previously. The goal with resistance training is to build muscle and strength.

Example:

Resistance Training				
DB Bench Press	5	12-15		90sec
Machine Chest Press	4	15-20		90sec
Cable Tricep Exstension	4	8-12		60 sec

This part of the program should take roughly 30 - 45 minutes to complete. Try to keep rest periods low but also listen to your body. If you feel you need more time in between sets then take it as needed.

After resistance training is a part labeled lifters choice. In appendix A, which is in the back of the book, you will find lists of exercises. Under "lifters choice" I will include muscle groups, as well as sets and rep ranges to use. This is meant for you to choose exercises you enjoy. If you enjoy bicep curls, or rows this is where you get to do them, if you have any energy left that is!

Lifters Choice - Chest, Triceps, Biceps				
	3	10-12		60 sec
	3	10-12		60 sec

This portion of the program is optional. I recommend doing the extra work because it is fun. You can try new things that may help you achieve your goals. But the main part of the training is the resistance training.

This last portion of the program is optional. Although it could be the most important. This is cardio, core and cooldown stretching. But what is cardio? Is it where you lift the weights faster? No, I'm just kidding. Cardio is any exercise that's primary goal is the increase of your heart rate, like running. But if you are like me, the only running you do is out of food or patience.

Despite widespread belief, cardio does not burn fat. It burns calories. The more calories you burn, the more fat you will burn. It is also great for maintaining healthy lungs and a healthy heart. I do recommend doing some cardio. In appendix A there will be a table including many cardio options for you to choose from, however, feel free to change it up. The key is to do at least 20-30 minutes of cardio to get your heart rate up and have you breathing heavily. You can also perform your cardio at the beginning of the workout if you prefer. I personally prefer to do it at the end and spend my energy on lifting, but I know some feel better completing cardio first.

The next portion to perform is the core exercises. These are designed to strengthen not only your abdominals, but your entire core. When most think of the core muscles they immediately think of the abdominal muscles. The core includes other muscles including your erectors in your back, your pelvic floor muscles, and your oblique muscles, as well as many other smaller muscles. These muscles are all used to keep us upright and protect our organs and our spine.

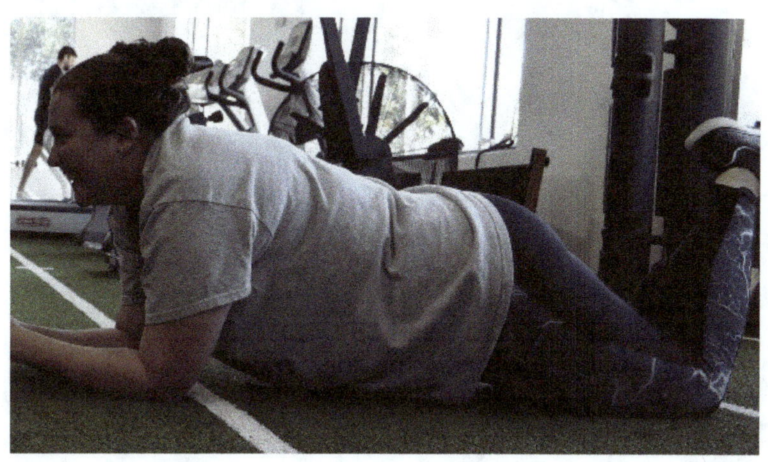

Static stretching is the last thing to do as part of your cooldown. This is your choice. Stretch however you feel, or wherever you feel you need to. The big key here is to hold each stretch for 30 seconds. Stretching is great for relaxing the muscles after strenuous activity. It can help the muscles recover and help with soreness the next day.

Cardio, Core, and Cool Down				
Cardio	n/a	n/a	n/a	n/a
Plank		2	30sec		60sec
Bird Dogs		2	8-12		60sec
Static Stretching	n/a	n/a	n/a	45 sec

PART 2

Chapter 5

Block 1

The first 4-week block will utilize mostly bodyweight, dumbbells, and machines. The goal of this block is to introduce you to the gym, and get you used to the movements that will continue throughout the program. We will also be building a solid base in which to grow from, introducing more advanced exercise and, modalities.

This block the number of movements is kept low. Each day will consist of mobility and activation followed by 3 movements. This is designed to make you familiar with the gym for the first few weeks without being overwhelmed. As you progress through each block, movements will be added to continue challenging you without overwhelming you. As always there will be a lifters choice adding additional movements if you choose.

Day 1 Bench Day -

Exercise	Sets	Reps	Weight	Rest Period
Mobility and Activation				
IYT Raises Chest Supported	2	6-8		45 sec
Dislocations	2	6-8		45 sec
Pushups	2	8-12		45 sec
Resistance Training				
DB Bench Press	5	12-15		90sec
Machine Chest Press	4	15-20		90sec
Cable Tricep Exstension	4	8-12		60 sec
Lifters Choice - Chest, Triceps, Biceps				
	3	10-12		60 sec
	3	10-12		60 sec
Cardio, Core, and Cool Down				
Cardio	n/a	n/a	n/a	n/a
Plank	2	30sec		60sec
Bird Dogs	2	8-12		60sec
Static Stretching	n/a	n/a	n/a	45 sec

Day 1 is **Bench Day**. First, you will start with **Mobility and Activation**. Set up a bench with roughly a 70-degree incline and use it to support the chest. Perform the IYT raises squeezing at the top and really trying to get your arms as far back as possible. This is going to help build the rotator muscles, the rear delt muscles, and warm the shoulders up. Follow this up by using either a pvc pipe or a band to perform dislocations. Finish with several sets of pushups. You can perform pushups from your knees, if necessary, but attempt a full pushup first. Until you have built enough strength to do a full push-up, start from your hands then drop to your knees when you can no longer perform full pushups.

Next is **Resistance Training**. This will begin with dumbbell bench press. Using dumbbells forces you to maintain tightness and control the weight. This helps to build the stabilization muscles as well as the chest and shoulders. You will follow this up with machine press. This can be either an actual machine that your gym has or a smith machine. The goal is to continue strengthening the chest and shoulders with more focus on those muscles rather than the stabilizers. You will then perform triceps extension to strengthen the arms.

The next part is **Lifters Choice**. Depending on how you are feeling, add an exercise you would like to try or that you enjoy. Appendix A will include a table from which to choose exercises.

Finally, you will finish the workout by completing **Cardio, Core, and Cooldown**. This portion of the program is optional but highly recommended. Cardio will help build your endurance as well as burn lots of calories, Core work is important for overall strength and posture. The cooldown will help to relax your muscles after strenuous activity.

<u>Day 2 Squat Day –</u>

Exercise	Sets	Reps	Weight	Rest Period
Mobility and Activation				
Kneeling hip exstensions	2	6-8		45 sec
Hip abduction and Adductions	2	8-12		45 sec
Bodyweight Lunges	2	8-12		45 sec
Resistance Training				
Paused Goblet Squats	5	8-12		90sec
Leg Exstensions	5	12-15		90sec
Bent over DB Rows	4	8-12		60 sec
Lifters Choice - Quads, Calves, Upper Back				
	3	10-12		60 sec
	3	10-12		60 sec
Cardio, Core, and Cool Down				
Cardio	n/a	n/a	n/a	n/a
Kettle Bell Swings	2	8-12		60 sec
Side Bends	2	12-15		60 sec
Static Stretching	n/a	n/a	n/a	45sec

Day 2 is **Squat Day**. First, you will start with **Mobility and Activation**. Beginning with hip extensions, you will start with one knee on the ground and the other forward with your foot planted with knee at a 90-degree angle. Push your hips forward trying to push your knee over your toe then return to starting position. Repeat with the other leg. Hip abductions and adductions can be done in several ways. If your gym has a machine feel free to use it. Otherwise, you can use a band or cable machine. Finally, you will perform some bodyweight lunges to finish warming up.

Next is **Resistance Training.** You will start with goblet squats. These are great for teaching proper squat technique. Adding in a pause will help to build confidence in the bottom of the squat which is the scariest part. If you have trouble hitting depth, you can elevate your heel on a plate or other items your gym may have. Leg extensions will help strengthen the quad muscles and bent over DB rows will help strengthen the back.

The next part is **Lifters Choice**. Depending on how you are feeling, add an exercise you would like to try or that you enjoy. Appendix A will include a table from which to choose exercises.

Finally, you will finish the workout by completing **Cardio, Core, and Cooldown**. This portion of the program is optional but highly recommended. Cardio will help build your endurance as well as burn lots of calories, Core work is important for overall strength and posture. The cooldown will help to relax your muscles after strenuous activity.

Day 3 Shoulders and Arms Day –

Exercise	Sets	Reps	Weight	Rest Period
Mobility and Activation				
External and Internal Shoulder Rotations	2	12-15		45 sec
DB overhead claps	2	8-12		45 sec
DB Reverse Flys	2	12-15		45 sec
Resistance Training				
Standing DB Overhead Press	5	12-15		90sec
Lateral Raises to front raises	3	8-12		90sec
Dips - assisted if necessary	4	12-15		60 sec
Lifters Choice - Delloids, triceps, Biceps				
	3	10-12		60 sec
	3	10-12		60 sec
Cardio, Core, and Cool Down				
Cardio	n/a	n/a	n/a	n/a
Cable Crunch	2	12-15		60 sec
Paloff Press	2	10-12		60 sec
Static Stretching	n/a	n/a	45 seconds	n/a

Day 3 begins is **Shoulders and Arms**. First, you will start with **Mobility and Activation.** Beginning with external and internal shoulder rotations. These can be done with a band or cable. Do not use a DB here. With your elbow tucked against your side and the band/cable in hand you will rotate your hand outward as far as your body will allow. Once the reps are completed you will use the other arm then repeat this exercise again, this time rotating your hands in towards your body. Next, while holding a DB in each hand bring your arms from your side to above your head and touch the backs of your hands. Use a light DB here. Finally finish with DB reverse flys. Simply bend forward at the waist with a DB in each hand and bring your hands out and back.

Resistance Training begins with standing DB press. This will strengthen your shoulders while also working your core and balance. It also forces you to maintain your brace and tightness while pressing. Follow up with side lateral raises and front raises. These are done together. You will perform the side raise followed by the front raise to equal 1 rep. You will finish up resistance training with dips. Dips can be performed assisted with a band or machine as needed.

The next part is **Lifters Choice**. Depending on how you are feeling, add in an exercise you would like to try or that you enjoy. Appendix A will include a table from which to choose exercises.

Finally, you will finish the workout by completing **Cardio, Core, and Cooldown**. This portion of the program is optional but highly recommended. Cardio will help build your endurance as well as burn lots of calories, Core work is important for overall strength and posture. The cooldown will help to relax your muscles after strenuous activity.

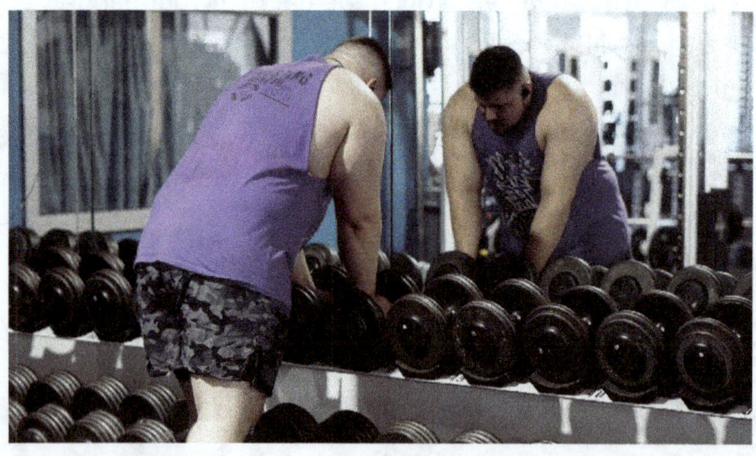

<u>Day 4 Deadlift Day –</u>

Exercise	Sets	Reps	Weight	Rest Period
Mobility and Activation				
Cat Cows	2	6-8		45 sec
Kneeling Kettle Bell Shifts	2	6-8		45 sec
Toe Touchdowns	2	8-12		45 sec
Resistance Training				
DB Romanian Deadlifts	5	8-12		90sec
Hamstring Curls	4	12-15		90sec
Pullups - Assisted if necessary	4	8-12		60 sec
Client Choice - Glutes, Hamstrings, Lats				
	3	10-12		60 sec
	3	10-12		60 sec
Cardio, Core, and Cool Down				
Cardio	n/a	n/a	n/a	n/a
Leg Lifts	2	8-12		60 sec
Mountain Climbers	2	12-15		60 sec
Static Stretching	n/a	n/a		45 seconds

Day 4 is **Deadlift Day.** First, you will start with **Mobility and Activation.** You will begin with cat cows. Staring on your hands and knees with a flat back you will arch your back as high as you can then do the opposite trying to touch your stomach to the ground. You will follow these with kneeling KB shifts. If you do not have access to a KB, a DB can be used. You will start on your knees. Take one leg and plant your foot pointing away from your body with your knee at a 90-degree angle. While holding the KB between your legs you will lean towards the planted leg as far as you can. Return to starting position. You will finish with toe touchdowns. Stack plates to your desired height. Stand with one foot on the stacked plates and the other foot hanging. Lower yourself and touch the ground and return to the start position.

Next you will perform **Resistance Training**. This will begin with DB Romanian deadlifts which will be the introduction to the hip hinge movement. This exercise will teach you the basic form needed for full deadlifts while also strengthening your hips and back. It will be followed by hamstring curls and finished up with pullups. Pullups can be assisted with a band or machine if necessary.

The next part is **Lifters Choice**. Depending on how you are feeling, add in an exercise you would like to try or that you enjoy. Appendix A will include a table from which to choose exercises.

Finally, you will finish the workout by completing **Cardio, Core, and Cooldown**. This portion of the program is optional but highly recommended. Cardio will help build your endurance as well as burn lots of calories, Core work is important for overall strength and posture. The cooldown will help to relax your muscles after strenuous activity.

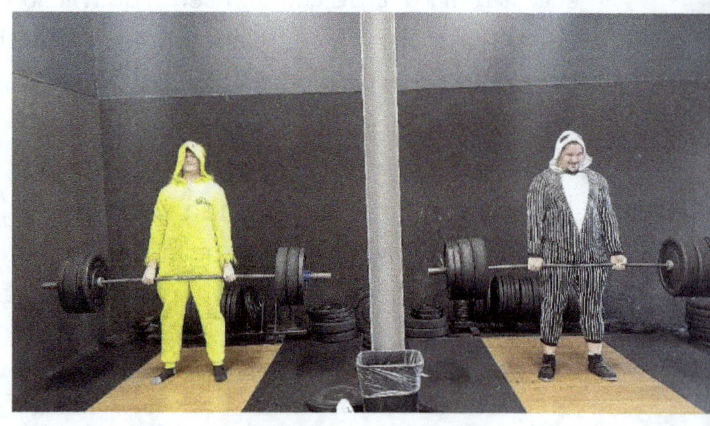

This finishes up one full week of training. You will perform the same exercises over the next two weeks, increasing the weight each week if possible. On the fourth week of training, you will perform a deload week. During the deload week, you will perform the same exercises but only for three sets. You will also use the lightest weight from week one for every set. This may seem redundant, but it allows your body to recover from the training before starting the next block and gives you a mental break to re-vitalize you before the next block.

Chapter 6
Block 2

The second 4-week block will continue and expand on what you learned in Block 1. With this block, we will introduce more unilateral exercises. This simply means you will be performing exercises on one side of the body, then the other. This will challenge your core and your balance and coordination. The goal of this block is to build on what you have learned, while continuing to grow and challenge you.

You will notice many of the same exercises, however the sets/reps have changed. This is to continue progressing the movements and making you stronger and more proficient in these movements. The number of exercises performed each day increased as well. After 4 weeks of lifting your body is getting used to working out and adding an additional movement will help continue your progress to achieve your goals.

<u>Day 1 Bench Day –</u>

Exercise	Sets	Reps	Weight	Rest Period
Mobility and Activation				
IYT Raises Chest Supported	2	6-8		45 sec
Dislocations	2	6-8		45 sec
Pushups	2	8-12		45 sec
Resistance Training				
Incline DB Bench Press - Alternating arm	5	8-12		90sec
Pec Flys	4	12-15		90sec
Dips - assisted if needed	5	8-12		60 sec
DB Skullcrushers	4	10-12		60sec
Lifters Choice - Chest, Triceps, Biceps				
	3	8-12		60 sec
	3	8-12		60 sec
	3	8-12		60 sec
Cardio, Core, and Cool Down				
Cardio	n/a	n/a	n/a	n/a
Plank	2	60sec		60sec
Bird Dogs	3	8-12		60sec
Static Stretching	n/a	n/a	n/a	45 sec

Day 1 is **Bench Day**. First, you will start with **Mobility and Activation**. This will be the same as Block 1.

Next is **Resistance Training**. This will begin with some alternating incline dumbbell bench press. You will perform the Incline DB press like normal, however you will only use one DB and perform one arm at a time. You will follow up with pec flys. This can be either a machine at your gym or continue using DB's. Whichever you choose, use that same exercise for the remainder of this block. The goal is to continue strengthening the chest, next you will perform dips. You will finish resistance training with some DB skull crushers.

The next part is **Lifters Choice**. Depending on how you are feeling, add in an exercise you would like to try or that you enjoy. Appendix A will include a table from which to choose exercises.

Finally, you will finish the workout by completing **Cardio, Core, and Cooldown**. This portion of the program is optional but highly recommended. Cardio will help build your endurance as well as burn lots of calories, Core work is important for overall strength and posture. The cooldown will help to relax your muscles after strenuous activity.

Day 2 Squat Day –

Exercise	Sets	Reps	Weight	Rest Period
Mobility and Activation				
Kneeling hip exstensions	2	6-8		45 sec
Elevated Touch downs	2	8-12		45 sec
Cosack Squats	2	8-12		45 sec
Resistance Training				
Cable Goblet Squats	5	8-12		90sec
Bulgarian Split Squats	3	8-12		90sec
Single Leg Leg Exstensions	4	12-15		60 sec
Chest Supported Incline DB Rows	5	12-15		60 sec
Lifters Choice - Quads, Calves, Upper Back				
	3	8-12		60 sec
	3	8-12		60 sec
	3	8-12		60 sec
Cardio, Core, and Cool Down				
Cardio	n/a	n/a	n/a	n/a
Russian Twists	2	8-12		60 sec
Side Bends	3	12-15		60 sec
Static Stretching	n/a	n/a	n/a	45sec

Day 2 is **Squat Day**. First, you will start with
Mobility and Activation. You will continue with kneeling
hip extension in this block. Abductions and adductions
have switched out for elevated touch downs. You
performed these on deadlift day last block. Lastly, you will
perform cossack squats. Stand with your feet wide. You
will squat sideways into one leg and back up to repeat on
your other side.

Next is **Resistance Training.** You will start with
cable goblet squats. With the cable goblet squat the
weight is pulling forward instead of down. This will force
you to engage your core more and focus on staying
upright. Next is the most hated exercise ever invented.
The Bulgarian split squats. With one foot elevated behind
you, bend your knee and squat. This may be difficult at
first with balance so stay close to something you can use
for assistance. Leg extensions will help strengthen the
quad muscles. This will be performed one leg at a time

instead of together this block. Lastly, the rows will help strengthen your back.

The next part is **Lifters Choice**. Depending on how you are feeling, add in an exercise you would like to try or that you enjoy. Appendix A will include a table from which to choose exercises.

Finally, you will finish the workout by completing **Cardio, Core, and Cooldown**. This portion of the program is optional but highly recommended. Cardio will help build your endurance as well as burn lots of calories, Core work is important for overall strength and posture. The cooldown will help to relax your muscles after strenuous activity.

Day 3 Shoulders and Arms Day –

Exercise	Sets	Reps	Weight	Rest Period
Mobility and Activation				
External and Internal Shoulder Rotations	2	12-15		45 sec
DB overhead claps	2	8-12		45 sec
DB Reverse Flys	3	12-15		45 sec
Resistance Training				
Seated Single Arm DB Press	5	8-12		90sec
Cable Lateral Raises	4	12-15		90sec
Single Arm Behind the neck Tricep Exstensions	5	12-15		60 sec
Cable Curls	5	12-15		60 sec
Lifters Choice - Deltoids, triceps, Biceps				
	3	8-12		60 sec
	3	8-12		60 sec
	3	8-12		60 sec
Cardio, Core, and Cool Down				
Cardio	n/a	n/a	n/a	n/a
Cable Crunch	2	12-15		60 sec
6 inches	3	60sec		60 sec
Static Stretching	n/a	n/a	45 seconds	n/a

Day 3 is **Shoulders and Arms**. First, you will start with **Mobility and Activation.** These will be the same as Block 1.

Resistance Training begins with seated single arm DB press. By performing the single arm variation, it will challenge your core and your balance. This allows you to train to improve imbalances such as one side being stronger than the other. Follow up with cable lateral raises. You will perform single arm DB tricep behind the neck tricep extensions. While standing hold a single DB above your head. Bend your arm and allow the DB to go behind your neck. Extend your arm back above your head. You will complete the resistance training with cable bicep curls.

The next part is **Lifters Choice**. Depending on how you are feeling, add in an exercise you would like to try or that you enjoy. Appendix A will include a table from which to choose exercises.

Finally, you will finish the workout by completing **Cardio, Core, and Cooldown**. This portion of the program is optional but highly recommended. Cardio will help build your endurance as well as burn lots of calories, Core work is important for overall strength and posture. The cooldown will help to relax your muscles after strenuous activity.

<u>Day 4 Deadlift Day –</u>

Exercise	Sets	Reps	Weight	Rest Period
Mobility and Activation				
Cat Cows	2	6-8		45 sec
Kneeling Kettle Bell Shifts	2	6-8		45 sec
Step ups	3	8-12		45 sec
Resistance Training				
DB Single Leg Romanian Deadlifts	5	8-12		90sec
Cable Pull throughs	4	12-15		90sec
Single Arm DB rows	5	8-12		60 sec
Pullups - Assisted if necessary	4	12-15		60 sec
Client Choice - Glutes, Hamstrings, Lats				
	3	8-12		60 sec
	3	8-12		60 sec
	3	8-12		60 sec
Cardio, Core, and Cool Down				
Cardio	n/a	n/a	n/a	n/a
Hanging Leg Lifts	2	8-12		60 sec
Mountain Climbers	3	12-15		60 sec
Static Stretching	n/a	n/a		45 seconds

Day 4 is **Deadlift Day.** First, you will start with **Mobility and Activation.** Toe touchdowns have been replaced with step ups. Find a box at a comfortable height and using one leg at a time step up onto the box and back down.

Next you will perform **Resistance Training**. This will begin with DB single leg Romanian deadlifts. Place one foot slightly behind you to use for balance. Perform single leg RDL's the same as normal except with one leg at a time. This will be followed by cable pull-throughs. Using a cable set low, stand facing away from the cable. Bend at the hips and reach through your legs to grab the cable. Squeeze your glutes and push your hips forward. Next perform the single arm DB row to strengthen your back. Finish with pullups. Pullups can be assisted with a band or machine if necessary.

The next part is **Lifters Choice**. Depending on how you are feeling, add in an exercise you would like to try or that you enjoy. Appendix A will include a table from which to choose exercises.

Finally, you will finish the workout by completing **Cardio, Core, and Cooldown**. This portion of the program is optional but highly recommended. Cardio will help build your endurance as well as burn lots of calories, Core work is important for overall strength and posture. The cooldown will help to relax your muscles after strenuous activity.

This finishes up one full week of training. You will perform the same exercises over the next two weeks, increasing the weight each week if possible. On the fourth week of training, you will perform a deload week. During the deload week, you will perform the same exercises but only for three sets. You will also use the lightest weight from week one for every set. This may seem redundant, but it allows your body to recover from the training before starting the next block and gives you a mental break to re-vitalize you before the next block.

Chapter 7

Block 3

We have now completed 8 weeks of training. Great Job! By now, you should have a good feel for your body, what you like and do not like, and exercises you should avoid due to pain, discomfort, or inability to perform. You may have lost a few pounds or gained some in muscle. You should have a good routine going regularly to the gym.

The next block begins to build on what you have already done. Barbell movements will be introduced into your training. One additional client choice exercise was added. You will perform more sets and reps during this block to really assess your endurance.

The barbell movements being introduced will be the squat, the bench press, and the deadlift. They will be performed in cluster sets. Do not let the 10 sets intimidate you. You should keep the weight light. I recommend using a weight that you can perform six to eight reps with. You should perform these sets with full attention on maintaining perfect form. Keep the rest times shorter than normal and make each set count. This will help to build technique and form as you move into later blocks of training and increase the intensity.

<u>Day 1 Bench Day –</u>

Exercise	Sets	Reps	Weight	Rest Period
Mobility and Activation				
IYT Raises Chest Supported	2	6-8		45 sec
Dislocations	2	6-8		45 sec
DB Bench press	2	25		45 sec
Resistance Training				
Bench Press	10	3		30 sec
DB Incline Bench	5	8-12		90 sec
Pec Flys - Paused	4	10-12		60 sec
Dips - assisted if necessary	2	AMAP		
Lifters Choice - Chest, Triceps, Biceps				
	3	12-15		60 sec
	3	12-15		60 sec
	3	12-15		60 sec
	3	12-15		60 sec
Cardio, Core, and Cool Down				
Cardio	n/a	n/a	n/a	n/a
Plank	3	ALAP		60sec
Mountain climbers	3	12-20		60sec
Static Stretching	n/a	n/a	n/a	45 sec

Day 1 is **Bench Day**. First, you will start with **Mobility and Activation**. The first 2 exercises will be the same as block 1. We have replaced pushups with DB bench press. You should use a very light weight and just focus on the movement.

Next is **Resistance Training**. This will begin with Bench Press. If you are still hesitant to do bench press, it is acceptable to use a smith machine. Do not let the 10 sets intimidate you. The weight should be light enough to perform 6-8 reps. The goal is to get under the bar, set up and perform 3 perfect reps. You will the perform DB incline bench. Follow this up with Pec flys. Pause at the peak of the flys and imagine your shoulders touching. Finish off with some dips.

The next part is **Lifters Choice**. Depending on how you are feeling, add in an exercise you would like to try or that you enjoy. Appendix A will include a table from which to choose exercises.

Finally, you will finish the workout by completing **Cardio, Core, and Cooldown**. This portion of the program is optional but highly recommended. Cardio will help build your endurance as well as burn lots of calories, Core work is important for overall strength and posture. The cooldown will help to relax your muscles after strenuous activity.

Day 2 Squat Day –

Exercise	Sets	Reps	Weight	Rest Period
Mobility and Activation				
Kneeling hip exstensions	2	6-8		45 sec
Elevated Touch downs	2	8-12		45 sec
Cosack Squats	2	8-12		45 sec
Resistance Training				
Squats	10	3		30 sec
Lunges	5	8-12		90 sec
Leg Exstensions + Leg Curls - Paused	3	12-15		60 sec
DB Chest Supported Rows	5	10-15		90 sec
Lifters Choice - Quads, Calves, Upper Back				
	3	12-15		60 sec
	3	12-15		60 sec
	3	12-15		60 sec
	3	12-15		60 sec
Cardio, Core, and Cool Down				
Cardio	n/a	n/a	n/a	n/a
Russian Twists	3	8-12		60 sec
Cable oblique twists	3	12-15		60 sec
Static Stretching	n/a	n/a	n/a	45sec

Day 2 is **Squat Day**. First, you will start with **Mobility and Activation**. This will be the same as the previous block.

Next is **Resistance Training.** This will begin with the Squat. Do not let the 10 sets intimidate you. The weight should be a weight you can perform for 6-8 reps. The goal is to perform 3 perfect reps. You can use any style of squat you want. This can be high bar, low bar, front squat, SSB squat, or even squats on a smith machine. Whatever you choose, use the same style for the remainder of the program. You will perform lunges. After the lunges you will perform a superset combo of leg extensions and curls. This simply means you will perform the leg extensions followed immediately by the curls, then rest.

The next part is **Lifters Choice**. Depending on how you are feeling, add in an exercise you would like to try or that you enjoy. Appendix A will include a table from which to choose exercises.

Finally, you will finish the workout by completing **Cardio, Core, and Cooldown**. This portion of the program is optional but highly recommended. Cardio will help build your endurance as well as burn lots of calories, Core work is important for overall strength and posture. The cooldown will help to relax your muscles after strenuous activity.

<u>Day 3 Shoulder and Arm Day –</u>

Exercise	Sets	Reps	Weight	Rest Period
Mobility and Activation				
External and Internal Shoulder Rotations	2	12-15		45 sec
DB Reverse Flys	3	8-12		45 sec
Standing DB Overhead press	2	25		45 sec
Resistance Training				
Seated Overhead Press	6	8-12		90 sec
DB Lateral Raises	5	8-12		90 sec
Tricep Exstensions	5	12-15		60 sec
Tempo DB Curls (0,2,5)	4	10-12		60 sec
Lifters Choice - Deltoids, triceps, Biceps				
	3	12-15		60 sec
	3	12-15		60 sec
	3	12-15		60 sec
	3	12-15		60 sec
Cardio, Core, and Cool Down				
Cardio	n/a	n/a	n/a	n/a
Cable Crunch	3	12-15		60 sec
6 inches	3	ALAP		60 sec
Static Stretching	n/a	n/a	45 seconds	n/a

Day 3 is **Shoulders and Arms**. First, start with **Mobility and Activation.** You will perform a standing DB overhead press instead of the overhead claps from the last block. Keep the weight very light.

Resistance Training will begin with a seated overhead press. If you cannot perform this with a barbell you should use a smith machine until you build up the strength to use a barbell. Next perform lateral raises with the DB, and tricep extensions. You will use the rope attachment on the cables. Keep your elbows tight to your side and try not to move them. Finally, you will perform a tempo DB curl.You will curl the weight up and squeeze your bicep for 2 seconds followed by a 5 second decent.

The next part is **Lifters Choice**. Depending on how you are feeling, add in an exercise you would like to try or that you enjoy. Appendix A will include a table from which to choose exercises.

Finally, you will finish the workout by completing **Cardio, Core, and Cooldown**. This portion of the program is optional but highly recommended. Cardio will help build your endurance as well as burn lots of calories, Core work is important for overall strength and posture. The cooldown will help to relax your muscles after strenuous activity.

<u>**Day 4 Deadlift Day –**</u>

Exercise	Sets	Reps	Weight	Rest Period
Mobility and Activation				
Cat Cows	2	6-8		45 sec
Kneeling Kettle Bell Shifts	2	6-8		45 sec
Step ups	3	8-12		45 sec
Resistance Training				
Romanian Deadlifts - BB	6	8-12		90 sec
Hip Thrusts	5	8-12		60 sec
DB Bent over Row	3	12-15		60 sec
Lat Pulldowns	5	12-15		60 sec
Client Choice - Glutes, Hamstrings, Lats				
	3	12-15		60 sec
	3	12-15		60 sec
	3	12-15		60 sec
	3	12-15		60 sec
Cardio, Core, and Cool Down				
Cardio	n/a	n/a	n/a	n/a
Hanging Leg Lifts	3	8-12		60 sec
Hyperexstensions	3	12-15		60 sec
Static Stretching	n/a	n/a		45 seconds

Day 4 is **Deadlift Day.** First, start with **Mobility and Activation.** This will be the same as the last block.

Next you will perform **Resistance Training**. This will begin with Romanian deadlifts with a BB and will be performed the same as with DB. Remember to keep the bar against your body and to hinge with the hips not the back. You will perform hip thrusts. If your gym has a dedicated machine for this movement use that. You will perform a DB bent over row and finish your resistance training with some lat pulldowns.

The next part is **Lifters Choice**. Depending on how you are feeling, add in an exercise you would like to try or that you enjoy. Appendix A will include a table from which to choose exercises.

Finally, you will finish the workout by completing **Cardio, Core, and Cooldown**. This portion of the program is optional but highly recommended. Cardio will help build your endurance as well as burn lots of calories, Core work is important for overall strength and posture. The cooldown will help to relax your muscles after strenuous activity.

This finishes up one full week of training. You will perform the same exercises over the next two weeks, increasing the weight each week if possible. On the fourth week of training, you will perform a deload week. During the deload week, you will perform the same exercises but only for three sets. You will also use the lightest weight from week one for every set. This may seem redundant, but it allows your body to recover from the training before starting the next block and gives you a mental break to re-vitalize you before the next block.

Chapter 8
Block 4

After 4 weeks of cluster sets, you should have a good feel for the main movements. Going forward you will continue to use these basic barbell movements. You will begin to increase weight to really challenge yourself.

This block will introduce tempo work. Introducing tempo work will force you to really feel the muscles through the entire movement. Tempo is a set speed at which you perform the exercise. For example, if the tempo is 5,2,0 then you would lower the weight for five seconds, pause for two seconds, then lift the weight as quickly as possible.

This block continues with challenging endurance. The reps will be high, combined with tempo work this block can be a bit brutal. Make sure to listen to your body and take adequate rest. This block will cause you to breathe heavily and sweat up a storm, so make sure you stay hydrated.

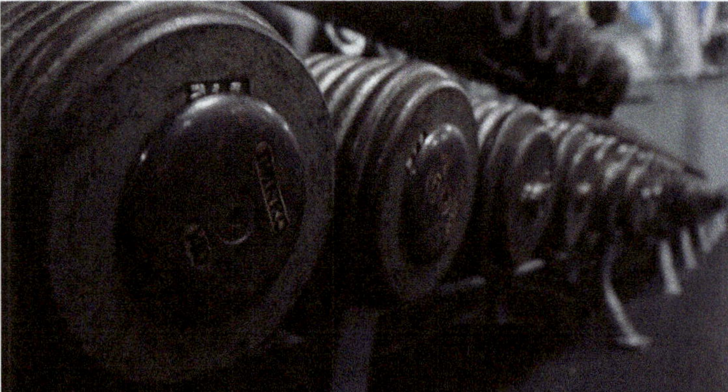

Day 1 Bench Day –

Exercise	Sets	Reps	Weight	Rest Period
Mobility and Activation				
IYT Raises Chest Supported	2	6-8		45 sec
Dislocations	2	6-8		45 sec
DB Bench press	2	25		45 sec
Resistance Training				
Bench Press	3	5-8		120 sec
DB Bench Press tempo (5.0.5)	5	12-15		90 sec
Dips - assisted if necessary	5	6-8		90 sec
Pushups	3	AMAP		
Lifters Choice - Chest. Triceps, Biceps				
	3	8-12		60 sec
	3	8-12		60 sec
	3	8-12		60 sec
	3	8-12		60 sec
Cardio, Core, and Cool Down				
Cardio	n/a	n/a	n/a	n/a
Ab wheel or BB rollout	3	6-12		60sec
Mountain climbers	3	12-20		60sec
Static Stretching	n/a	n/a	n/a	45 sec

Day 1 is **Bench Day**. First, start with **Mobility and Activation**. This will be the same as the last block.

Next is **Resistance Training**. This will begin with Bench Press. If you are still hesitant to do bench press it is acceptable to use a smith machine. You will perform 5 to 8 reps each set. If you manage 8 reps increase the weight by 5lbs. Once you can only perform 5 reps, do not increase the weight any further. Your goal is to beat that weight by week 3 of this block. You will perform DB bench press with a tempo. 5 seconds down, no pause, then 5 seconds up with no pause again. Next, you will perform dips. If you cannot accomplish bodyweight dips, or you are too fatigued from previous exercises then perform them assisted. You will finish with pushups by performing 3 sets to absolute failure. Each week your goal should be to beat each sets reps by 1.

The next part is **Lifters Choice**. Depending on how you are feeling, add in an exercise you would like to try or that you enjoy. Appendix A will include a table from which to choose exercises.

Finally, you will finish the workout by completing **Cardio, Core, and Cooldown**. This portion of the program is optional but highly recommended. Cardio will help build your endurance as well as burn lots of calories, Core work is important for overall strength and posture. The cooldown will help to relax your muscles after strenuous activity.

Day 2 Squat Day –

Exercise	Sets	Reps	Weight	Rest Period
Mobility and Activation				
Kneeling hip exstensions	2	6-8		45 sec
Elevated Touch downs	2	8-12		45 sec
Cosack Squats	2	8-12		45 sec
Resistance Training				
Squats	3	5-8		120 sec
Hack Squat paused	5	8-12		90 sec
Leg Exstensions Tempo (5,0,5)	4	8-12		90 sec
Cable Row Tempo (0,3,5)	5	10-12		120 sec
Lifters Choice - Quads, Calves, Upper Back				
	3	8-12		60 sec
	3	8-12		60 sec
	3	8-12		60 sec
	3	8-12		60 sec
Cardio, Core, and Cool Down				
Cardio	n/a	n/a	n/a	n/a
Hanging Leg Lifts	3	8-12		60 sec
Landmine Oblique twists	3	12-15		60 sec
Static Stretching	n/a	n/a	n/a	45sec

Day 2 is **Squat Day**. First, start with **Mobility and Activation**. These will be the same as previous block.

Next is **Resistance Training.** This will begin with the Squat. You will perform 5 to 8 reps each set. If you complete 8 reps, increase the weight by 5lbs. When you can only perform 5 reps <u>do not</u> increase the weight any further. Your goal is to beat that weight by week 3 of this block. Next perform the hack squat with a pause at the bottom. If your gym does not have a hack squat, use a leg press or a goblet squat. Perform leg extensions with a tempo. 5 seconds down, no pause, then 5 seconds up with no pause and finish with tempo cable row. Row the weight to you and pause for 3 seconds, and control the weight back with a 5 second eccentric.

The next part is **Lifters Choice**. Depending on how you are feeling, add in an exercise you would like to try or that you enjoy. Appendix A will include a table from which to choose exercises.

Finally, you will finish the workout by completing **Cardio, Core, and Cooldown**. This portion of the program is optional but highly recommended. Cardio will help build your endurance as well as burn lots of calories, Core work is important for overall strength and posture. The cooldown will help to relax your muscles after strenuous activity.

Day 3 Shoulder and Arm Day –

Exercise	Sets	Reps	Weight	Rest Period
Mobility and Activation				
External and Internal Shoulder Rotations	2	12-15		45 sec
DB Reverse Flys	3	8-12		45 sec
Standing DB Overhead press	2	25		45 sec
Resistance Training				
Arnold Press	5	8-12		90 sec
Upright Row	4	10-14		90 sec
DB Rolling Tricep Exstensions	5	12-15		60 sec
Eccentric Preacher Curls Tempo (0,0,5)	3	6-8		120 sec
Lifters Choice - Deltoids, triceps, Biceps				
	3	8-12		60 sec
	3	8-12		60 sec
	3	8-12		60 sec
	3	8-12		60 sec
Cardio, Core, and Cool Down				
Cardio	n/a	n/a	n/a	n/a
Crunches	1	100		
Side Planks	3	60 sec		60 sec
Static Stretching	n/a	n/a	45 seconds	n/a

Day 3 is **Shoulders and Arms**. First, start with
Mobility and Activation. This will be the same as the
previous block.

Resistance Training will begin with the Arnold
Press. You will perform these standing. With a DB in each
hand starting with your hands in front of you, bring your
arms out and press above your head then return to the
starting position. Next perform upright rows. Using a bar,
hold the bar at your hips, then bring the bar up to your
chin. Then perform rolling DB tricep extensions. Lying on
your back hold a DB in each hand. Bring the DB down to
your shoulders and press them back up. Finally, perform
the preacher curl with an eccentric focused tempo. Star at
the top and slowly lower the weight with a 5 second
lowering. Lift the weight back to the top and repeat the 5
second lowering.

The next part is the **Lifters Choice**. Depending on
how you are feeling, add in an exercise you would like to

try or that you enjoy. Appendix A will include a table from which to choose exercises.

Finally, you will finish the workout by completing **Cardio, Core, and Cooldown**. This portion of the program is optional but highly recommended. Cardio will help build your endurance as well as burn lots of calories, Core work is important for overall strength and posture. The cooldown will help to relax your muscles after strenuous activity.

<u>Day 4 Deadlift Day –</u>

Exercise	Sets	Reps	Weight	Rest Period
Mobility and Activation				
Cat Cows	2	6-8		45 sec
Kneeling Kettle Bell Shifts	2	6-8		45 sec
Step ups	3	8-12		45 sec
Resistance Training				
Deadlifts	10	3		30 sec
Nordic Curls Tempo (5,0,0)	5	8-12		90 sec
Single Arm Rows	4	10-15		90 sec
Pullups assisted if necassary	3	AMAP		
Client Choice - Glutes, Hamstrings, Lats				
	3	8-12		60 sec
	3	8-12		60 sec
	3	8-12		60 sec
	3	8-12		60 sec
Cardio, Core, and Cool Down				
Cardio	n/a	n/a	n/a	n/a
Glute Bridge March	3	8-12		60 sec
Hyperexstensions	3	12-15		60 sec
Static Stretching	n/a	n/a		45 seconds

Day 4 is **Deadlift Day.** First, start with **Mobility and Activation.** This will be the same as the last block.

Next up you will perform the **Resistance Training.** You will begin with Deadlifts. For this block perform deadlifts as a cluster set like you did for the other lifts in the previous block. You will perform Nordic curls with a tempo. You simply lower your body with a 5 second eccentric. You can use your hands to get back up if you need. Next perform single arm rows and finish with pullups. If you are unable to perform more than 5 pullups use assistance. You will perform 3 sets to absolute failure. Each week your goal is to beat each sets reps by 1.

The next part is **Lifters Choice.** Depending on how you are feeling, add in an exercise you would like to try or that you enjoy. Appendix A will include a table from which to choose exercises.

Finally, you will finish the workout by completing **Cardio, Core, and Cooldown**. This portion of the program is optional but highly recommended. Cardio will help build your endurance as well as burn lots of calories, Core work is important for overall strength and posture. The cooldown will help to relax your muscles after strenuous activity.

This finishes up one full week of training. You will perform the same exercises over the next two weeks, increasing the weight each week if possible. On the fourth week of training, you will perform a deload week. During the deload week, you will perform the same exercises but only for three sets. You will also use the lightest weight from week one for every set. This may seem redundant, but it allows your body to recover from the training before starting the next block and gives you a mental break to re-vitalize you before the next block.

Chapter 9

Block 5

This block of training will focus on strength. The reps will be lower, but the weight should be higher. Your focus for this block is to really push yourself to see where you are as far as strength goes. This block is not a powerlifting block. It is simply designed to increase your strength before moving back to more endurance or stabilization work. You will not be attempting any one rep maxes for this block and will stay in the 3-5 rep range to improve your strength.

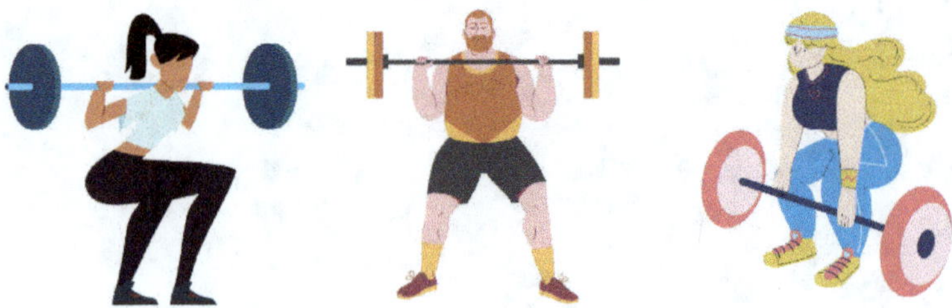

Day 1 Bench Day –

Exercise	Sets	Reps	Weight	Rest Period
Mobility and Activation				
IYT Raises Chest Supported	2	6-8		45 sec
Dislocations	2	6-8		45 sec
DB Bench press	2	25		45 sec
Resistance Training				
Bench Press	3	3-5		120 sec
Paused Bench Press	6	3	80% of heavisest bench that day	45 sec
Pec Flys	5	6-10		90 sec
JM Press	4	6-8		
Lifters Choice - Chest, Triceps, Biceps				
	3	8-10		60 sec
	3	8-10		60 sec
	3	8-10		60 sec
	3	8-10		60 sec
Cardio, Core, and Cool Down				
Cardio	n/a	n/a	n/a	n/a
Ab wheel or BB rollout	3	12-15		60sec
Eccentric Decline Situps Tempo (0.0.5)	3	8-12		60sec
Static Stretching	n/a	n/a	n/a	45 sec

Day 1 is **Bench Day**. First, start with **Mobility and Activation**. This will be the same as the last block.

Next is **Resistance Training**. This will begin with Bench Press. If you are still hesitant to do bench press use a smith machine. You will perform 3 to 5 reps on each set. If you manage 5 reps increase the weight by 5lbs. Once you can only perform 3 reps do not increase the weight any further. Your goal is to beat that weight by week 3 of this block. After you perform your heaviest bench for the day, you will lower the weight to 80% of the heaviest weight you used that day. You will perform 6 sets of 3 reps paused. Focus on moving the weight as fast as possible. Then perform pec flys and finish with JM press.

The next part is the **Lifters Choice**. Depending on how you are feeling, add in an exercise you would like to try or that you enjoy. Appendix A will include a table from which to choose exercises.

Finally, you will finish the workout by completing **Cardio, Core, and Cooldown**. This portion of the program is optional but highly recommended. Cardio will help build your endurance as well as burn lots of calories, Core work is important for overall strength and posture. The cooldown will help to relax your muscles after strenuous activity.

<u>Day 2 Squat Day –</u>

Exercise	Sets	Reps	Weight	Rest Period
Mobility and Activation				
Kneeling hip exstensions	2	6-8		45 sec
Elevated Touch downs	2	8-12		45 sec
Cosack Squats	2	8-12		45 sec
Resistance Training				
Squats	3	3-5		120 sec
Paused Squats	6	3	80% of heaviest squat that day	45 sec
DB RDL	4	8-12		60 sec
Landmine Rows	5	8-12		90 sec
Lifters Choice - Quads, Calves, Upper Back				
	3	8-10		60 sec
	3	8-10		60 sec
	3	8-10		60 sec
	3	8-10		60 sec
Cardio, Core, and Cool Down				
Cardio	n/a	n/a	n/a	n/a
Hanging Leg Lifts	3	8-12		60 sec
Landmine Oblique twists	3	12-15		60 sec
Static Stretching	n/a	n/a	n/a	45sec

Day 2 is **Squat Day**. First, start with **Mobility and Activation**. These will be the same as previous block.

Next is **Resistance Training.** This will begin with the Squat. You will perform 3 to 5 reps on each set. If you manage 5 reps increase the weight by 5lbs. Once you can only perform 3 reps do not increase the weight any further. Your goal is to beat that weight by week 3 of this block. After you perform your heaviest Squat for the day you will lower the weight to 80% of the heaviest weight you used that day. You will perform 6 sets of 3 reps paused. Focus on moving the weight as fast as possible. You will perform DB RDLs and finish with landmine rows.

The next part is **Lifters Choice**. Depending on how you are feeling, add in an exercise you would like to try or that you enjoy. Appendix A will include a table from which to choose exercises.

Finally, you will finish the workout by completing **Cardio, Core, and Cooldown**. This portion of the program is optional but highly recommended. Cardio will help build your endurance as well as burn lots of calories, Core work is important for overall strength and posture. The cooldown will help to relax your muscles after strenuous activity.

Day 3 Shoulders and Arms Day –

Exercise	Sets	Reps	Weight	Rest Period
Mobility and Activation				
External and Internal Shoulder Rotations	2	12-15		45 sec
DB Reverse Flys	3	8-12		45 sec
Standing DB Overhead press	2	25		45 sec
Resistance Training				
Seated Overhead Press	5	6-8		120 sec
Seated DB Lateral Raises	4	8-12		90 sec
Skullcrushers	5	8-12		90 sec
Swinging Hammer Curls	4	6-8		120 sec
Lifters Choice - Deltoids, triceps, Biceps				
	3	8-10		60 sec
	3	8-10		60 sec
	3	8-10		60 sec
	3	8-10		60 sec
Cardio, Core, and Cool Down				
Cardio	n/a	n/a	n/a	n/a
Crunches - Paused	4	25		
Suitcase Carries - heavy	3	50 ft		60 sec
Static Stretching	n/a	n/a	n/a	45 seconds

Day 3 is **Shoulders and Arms**. First, start with **Mobility and Activation.** You will perform a standing DB overhead press instead of the overhead claps from the last block. Keep the weight very light.

Resistance Training will begin with a seated overhead press. If you cannot perform this with a barbell, you should use a smith machine until you can build up the strength to use a barbell. Next, perform seated lateral raises with the DB and then perform skull crushers. Bring the bar towards your eyes while keeping your elbows tight and unmoving. Finally, perform swinging hammer curls. Do not worry about strict form. Focus on keeping your elbows from moving while swinging the weight up.

The next part is **Lifters Choice**. Depending on how you are feeling, add in an exercise you would like to try or that you enjoy. Appendix A will include a table from which to choose exercises.

Finally, you will finish the workout by completing **Cardio, Core, and Cooldown**. This portion of the program is optional but highly recommended. Cardio will help build your endurance as well as burn lots of calories, Core work is important for overall strength and posture. The cooldown will help to relax your muscles after strenuous activity.

Day 4 Deadlift Day –

Exercise	Sets	Reps	Weight	Rest Period
Mobility and Activation				
Cat Cows	2	6-8		45 sec
Kneeling Kettle Bell Shifts	2	6-8		45 sec
Step ups	3	8-12		45 sec
Resistance Training				
Deadlifts	3	4-6		120 sec
Deadlifts - Speed	6	3	80% of heaviest deadlift that day	90 sec
Incline Chest supported rows	4	6-8		90 sec
Lat Pulldowns - Tempo (0,2,5)	5	8-12		
Client Choice - Glutes, Hamstrings, Lats				
	3	8-10		60 sec
	3	8-10		60 sec
	3	8-10		60 sec
	3	8-10		60 sec
Cardio, Core, and Cool Down				
Cardio	n/a	n/a	n/a	n/a
Superman - Paused	3	12-15		60 sec
Kettlebell Bridge Pullover	3	8-12		60 sec
Static Stretching	n/a	n/a		45 seconds

Day 4 is **Deadlift Day.** First, start with **Mobility and Activation.** This will be the same as the last block.

Next you will perform the **Resistance Training**. You will begin with Deadlifts. For this block, you will perform heavier deadlifts. By this point your deadlift technique should be locked in. Push your limits and see how heavy you can lift for 4 to 6 reps. After you perform your heaviest deadlift for the day lower the weight to 80% of the heaviest weight you used that day. Perform 6 sets of 3 reps. Focus on exploding, moving the bar fast. You will perform incline chest supported rows and finish with lat pulldowns with a tempo. Pull the weight down, pause for 2 seconds then slowly let the weight back up with a 5 second eccentric.

The next part is **Lifters Choice**. Depending on how you are feeling, add in an exercise you would like to try or that you enjoy. Appendix A will include a table from which to choose exercises.

Finally, you will finish the workout by completing **Cardio, Core, and Cooldown**. This portion of the program is optional but highly recommended. Cardio will help build your endurance as well as burn lots of calories, Core work is important for overall strength and posture. The cooldown will help to relax your muscles after strenuous activity.

This finishes up one full week of training. You will perform the same exercises over the next two weeks, increasing the weight each week if possible. On the fourth week of training, you will perform a deload week. During the deload week, you will perform the same exercises but only for three sets. You will also use the lightest weight from week one for every set. This may seem redundant, but it allows your body to recover from the training before starting the next block and gives you a mental break to re-vitalize you before the next block.

By the end of this block, you should have a three-rep max in each of your lifts. You can find a one rep max calculator online and put the numbers in to get a rough estimate of your one rep max.

This concludes the 20-week program. From this point this program can be repeated for another 20 weeks. Simply change the choices and do different exercises. You can also switch your squat, bench, and deadlift technique for a different one. If you do not want to re-run this program another program can be found for a more intermediate level of training. By this point you should have a good idea of what type of training you enjoy.

Look for more of my books, coming soon, including other variations of days and more intermediate level and eventually advanced level programs.

The achievement of one goal should be the starting point of another!

Chapter 10
Full Program

For this chapter you will have the program laid out including a section for weight. You can use this to track your weight as you progress through the program. There are a few ways to do this.

1. Scan the pages and place them in a notebook.
2. Take a picture with your phone, using edit write the weight in.
3. Write everything in a notebook.
4. Simply write in this book. You bought it after all!

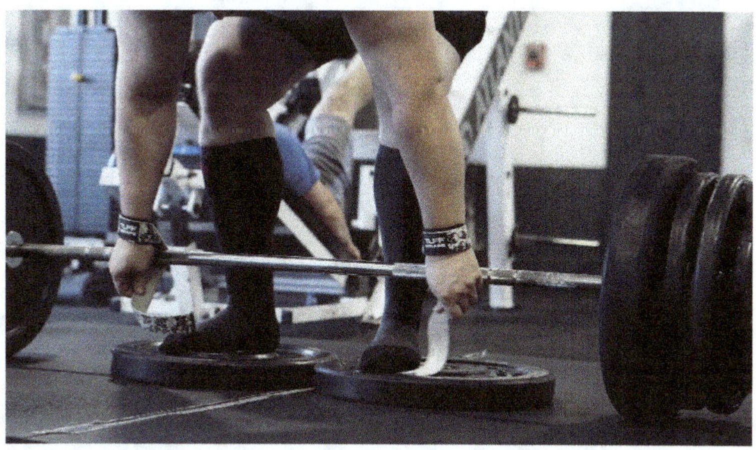

Block 1

(Repeat for 3 weeks, then deload)

Exercise	Sets	Reps	Weight	Rest Period
Mobility and Activation				
IYT Raises Chest Supported	2	6-8		45 sec
Dislocations	2	6-8		45 sec
Pushups	2	8-12		45 sec
Resistance Training				
DB Bench Press	5	12-15		90sec
Machine Chest Press	4	15-20		90sec
Cable Tricep Exstension	4	8-12		60 sec
Lifters Choice - Chest, Triceps, Biceps				
	3	10-12		60 sec
	3	10-12		60 sec
Cardio, Core, and Cool Down				
Cardio	n/a	n/a	n/a	n/a
Plank	2	30sec		60sec
Bird Dogs	2	8-12		60sec
Static Stretching	n/a	n/a	n/a	45 sec

Exercise	Sets	Reps	Weight	Rest Period
Mobility and Activation				
Kneeling hip exstensions	2	6-8		45 sec
Hip abduction and Adductions	2	8-12		45 sec
Bodyweight Lunges	2	8-12		45 sec
Resistance Training				
Paused Goblet Squats	5	8-12		90sec
Leg Exstensions	5	12-15		90sec
Bent over DB Rows	4	8-12		60 sec
Lifters Choice - Quads, Calves, Upper Back				
	3	10-12		60 sec
	3	10-12		60 sec
Cardio, Core, and Cool Down				
Cardio	n/a	n/a	n/a	n/a
Kettle Bell Swings	2	8-12		60 sec
Side Bends	2	12-15		60 sec
Static Stretching	n/a	n/a	n/a	45sec

Exercise	Sets	Reps	Weight	Rest Period
Mobility and Activation				
External and Internal Shoulder Rotations	2	12-15		45 sec
DB overhead claps	2	8-12		45 sec
DB Reverse Flys	2	12-15		45 sec
Resistance Training				
Standing DB Overhead Press	5	12-15		90sec
Lateral Raises to front raises	3	8-12		90sec
Dips - assisted if necessary	4	12-15		60 sec
Lifters Choice - Deltoids, triceps, Biceps				
	3	10-12		60 sec
	3	10-12		60 sec
Cardio, Core, and Cool Down				
Cardio	n/a	n/a	n/a	n/a
Cable Crunch	2	12-15		60 sec
Paloff Press	2	10-12		60 sec
Static Stretching	n/a	n/a	45 seconds	n/a

Exercise	Sets	Reps	Weight	Rest Period
Mobility and Activation				
Cat Cows	2	6-8		45 sec
Kneeling Kettle Bell Shifts	2	6-8		45 sec
Toe Touchdowns	2	8-12		45 sec
Resistance Training				
DB Romanian Deadlifts	5	8-12		90sec
Hamstring Curls	4	12-15		90sec
Pullups - Assisted if necessary	4	8-12		60 sec
Client Choice - Glutes, Hamstrings, Lats				
	3	10-12		60 sec
	3	10-12		60 sec
Cardio, Core, and Cool Down				
Cardio	n/a	n/a	n/a	n/a
Leg Lifts	2	8-12		60 sec
Mountain Climbers	2	12-15		60 sec
Static Stretching	n/a	n/a		45 seconds

Block 2

(Repeat for 3 weeks, then deload)

Exercise	Sets	Reps	Weight	Rest Period
Mobility and Activation				
IYT Raises Chest Supported	2	6-8		45 sec
Dislocations	2	6-8		45 sec
Pushups	2	8-12		45 sec
Resistance Training				
Incline DB Bench Press - Alternating arm	5	8-12		90sec
Pec Flys	4	12-15		90sec
Dips - assisted if needed	5	8-12		60 sec
DB Skullcrushers	4	10-12		60sec
Lifters Choice - Chest, Triceps, Biceps				
	3	8-12		60 sec
	3	8-12		60 sec
	3	8-12		60 sec
Cardio, Core, and Cool Down				
Cardio	n/a	n/a	n/a	n/a
Plank	2	60sec		60sec
Bird Dogs	3	8-12		60sec
Static Stretching	n/a	n/a	n/a	45 sec

Exercise	Sets	Reps	Weight	Rest Period
Mobility and Activation				
Kneeling hip exstensions	2	6-8		45 sec
Elevated Touch downs	2	8-12		45 sec
Cosack Squats	2	8-12		45 sec
Resistance Training				
Cable Goblet Squats	5	8-12		90sec
Bulgarian Split Squats	3	8-12		90sec
Single Leg Leg Exstensions	4	12-15		60 sec
Chest Supported Incline DB Rows	5	12-15		60 sec
Lifters Choice - Quads, Calves, Upper Back				
	3	8-12		60 sec
	3	8-12		60 sec
	3	8-12		60 sec
Cardio, Core, and Cool Down				
Cardio	n/a	n/a	n/a	n/a
Russian Twists	2	8-12		60 sec
Side Bends	3	12-15		60 sec
Static Stretching	n/a	n/a	n/a	45sec

Exercise	Sets	Reps	Weight	Rest Period
Mobility and Activation				
External and Internal Shoulder Rotations	2	12-15		45 sec
DB overhead claps	2	8-12		45 sec
DB Reverse Flys	3	12-15		45 sec
Resistance Training				
Seated Single Arm DB Press	5	8-12		90sec
Cable Lateral Raises	4	12-15		90sec
Single Arm Behind the neck Tricep Exstensions	5	12-15		60 sec
Cable Curls	5	12-15		60 sec
Lifters Choice - Deltoids, triceps, Biceps				
	3	8-12		60 sec
	3	8-12		60 sec
	3	8-12		60 sec
Cardio, Core, and Cool Down				
Cardio	n/a	n/a	n/a	n/a
Cable Crunch	2	12-15		60 sec
6 inches	3	60sec		60 sec
Static Stretching	n/a	n/a	45 seconds	n/a

Exercise	Sets	Reps	Weight	Rest Period
Mobility and Activation				
Cat Cows	2	6-8		45 sec
Kneeling Kettle Bell Shifts	2	6-8		45 sec
Step ups	3	8-12		45 sec
Resistance Training				
DB Single Leg Romanian Deadlifts	5	8-12		90sec
Cable Pull throughs	4	12-15		90sec
Single Arm DB rows	5	8-12		60 sec
Pullups - Assisted if necessary	4	12-15		60 sec
Client Choice - Glutes, Hamstrings, Lats				
	3	8-12		60 sec
	3	8-12		60 sec
	3	8-12		60 sec
Cardio, Core, and Cool Down				
Cardio	n/a	n/a	n/a	n/a
Hanging Leg Lifts	2	8-12		60 sec
Mountain Climbers	3	12-15		60 sec
Static Stretching	n/a	n/a		45 seconds

Block 3

(Repeat for 3 weeks, then deload)

Exercise	Sets	Reps	Weight	Rest Period
Mobility and Activation				
IYT Raises Chest Supported	2	6-8		45 sec
Dislocations	2	6-8		45 sec
DB Bench press	2	25		45 sec
Resistance Training				
Bench Press	10	3		30 sec
DB Incline Bench	5	8-12		90 sec
Pec Flys - Paused	4	10-12		60 sec
Dips - assisted if necessary	2	AMAP		
Lifters Choice - Chest, Triceps, Biceps				
	3	12-15		60 sec
	3	12-15		60 sec
	3	12-15		60 sec
	3	12-15		60 sec
Cardio, Core, and Cool Down				
Cardio	n/a	n/a	n/a	n/a
Plank	3	ALAP		60sec
Mountain climbers	3	12-20		60sec
Static Stretching	n/a	n/a	n/a	45 sec

Exercise	Sets	Reps	Weight	Rest Period
Mobility and Activation				
Kneeling hip exstensions	2	6-8		45 sec
Elevated Touch downs	2	8-12		45 sec
Cossack Squats	2	8-12		45 sec
Resistance Training				
Squats	10	3		30 sec
Lunges	5	8-12		90 sec
Leg Extensions + Leg Curls - Paused	3	12-15		60 sec
DB Chest Supported Rows	5	10-15		90 sec
Lifters Choice - Quads, Calves, Upper Back				
	3	12-15		60 sec
	3	12-15		60 sec
	3	12-15		60 sec
	3	12-15		60 sec
Cardio, Core, and Cool Down				
Cardio	n/a	n/a	n/a	n/a
Russian Twists	3	8-12		60 sec
Cable oblique twists	3	12-15		60 sec
Static Stretching	n/a	n/a	n/a	45sec

Exercise	Sets	Reps	Weight	Rest Period
Mobility and Activation				
External and Internal Shoulder Rotations	2	12-15		45 sec
DB Reverse Flys	2	8-12		45 sec
Standing DB Overhead press	2	25		45 sec
Resistance Training				
Seated Overhead Press	6	8-12		90 sec
DB Lateral Raises	5	8-12		90 sec
Tricep Exstensions	5	12-15		60 sec
Tempo DB Curls (0,2,5)	4	10-12		60 sec
Lifters Choice - Deltoids, triceps, Biceps				
	3	12-15		60 sec
	3	12-15		60 sec
	3	12-15		60 sec
	3	12-15		60 sec
Cardio, Core, and Cool Down				
Cardio	n/a	n/a	n/a	n/a
Cable Crunch	3	12-15		60 sec
6 inches	3	ALAP		60 sec
Static Stretching	n/a	n/a	45 seconds	n/a

Exercise	Sets	Reps	Weight	Rest Period
Mobility and Activation				
Cat Cows	2	6-8		45 sec
Kneeling Kettle Bell Shifts	2	6-8		45 sec
Step ups	3	8-12		45 sec
Resistance Training				
Romanian Deadlifts - BB	6	8-12		90 sec
Hip Thrusts	5	8-12		60 sec
DB Bent over Row	3	12-15		60 sec
Lat Pulldowns	5	12-15		60 sec
Client Choice - Glutes, Hamstrings, Lats				
	3	12-15		60 sec
	3	12-15		60 sec
	3	12-15		60 sec
	3	12-15		60 sec
Cardio, Core, and Cool Down				
Cardio	n/a	n/a	n/a	n/a
Hanging Leg Lifts	3	8-12		60 sec
Hyperexstensions	3	12-15		60 sec
Static Stretching	n/a	n/a		45 seconds

Block 4

(Repeat for 3 weeks, then deload)

Exercise	Sets	Reps	Weight	Rest Period
Mobility and Activation				
IYT Raises Chest Supported	2	6-8		45 sec
Dislocations	2	6-8		45 sec
DB Bench press	2	25		45 sec
Resistance Training				
Bench Press	3	5-8		120 sec
DB Bench Press tempo (5,0,5)	5	12-15		90 sec
Dips - assisted if necessary	5	6-8		90 sec
Pushups	3	AMAP		
Lifters Choice - Chest, Triceps, Biceps				
	3	8-12		60 sec
	3	8-12		60 sec
	3	8-12		60 sec
	3	8-12		60 sec
Cardio, Core, and Cool Down				
Cardio	n/a	n/a	n/a	n/a
Ab wheel or BB rollout	3	8-12		60sec
Mountain climbers	3	12-20		60sec
Static Stretching	n/a	n/a	n/a	45 sec

Exercise	Sets	Reps	Weight	Rest Period
Mobility and Activation				
Kneeling hip exstensions	2	6-8		45 sec
Elevated Touch downs	2	8-12		45 sec
Cosack Squats	2	8-12		45 sec
Resistance Training				
Squats	3	5-8		120 sec
Hack Squat paused	5	8-12		90 sec
Leg Exstensions Tempo (5,0,5)	4	8-12		90 sec
Cable Row Tempo (0,3,5)	5	10-12		120 sec
Lifters Choice - Quads, Calves, Upper Back				
	3	8-12		60 sec
	3	8-12		60 sec
	3	8-12		60 sec
	3	8-12		60 sec
Cardio, Core, and Cool Down				
Cardio	n/a	n/a	n/a	n/a
Hanging Leg Lifts	3	8-12		60 sec
Landmine Oblique twists	3	12-15		60 sec
Static Stretching	n/a	n/a	n/a	45sec

Exercise	Sets	Reps	Weight	Rest Period
Mobility and Activation				
External and Internal Shoulder Rotations	2	12-15		45 sec
DB Reverse Flys	3	8-12		45 sec
Standing DB Overhead press	2	25		45 sec
Resistance Training				
Arnold Press	5	8-12		90 sec
Upright Row	4	10-14		90 sec
DB Rolling Tricep Exstensions	5	12-15		60 sec
Eccentric Preacher Curls Tempo (0,0,5)	3	6-8		120 sec
Lifters Choice - Deltoids, triceps, Biceps				
	3	8-12		60 sec
	3	8-12		60 sec
	3	8-12		60 sec
	3	8-12		60 sec
Cardio, Core, and Cool Down				
Cardio	n/a	n/a	n/a	n/a
Crunches	1	100		
Side Planks	3	60 sec		60 sec
Static Stretching	n/a	n/a	45 seconds	n/a

Exercise	Sets	Reps	Weight	Rest Period
Mobility and Activation				
Cat Cows	2	6-8		45 sec
Kneeling Kettle Bell Shifts	2	6-8		45 sec
Step ups	3	8-12		45 sec
Resistance Training				
Deadlifts	10	3		30 sec
Nordic Curls Tempo (5,0,0)	5	8-12		90 sec
Single Arm Rows	4	10-15		90 sec
Pullups assisted if necassary	3 AMAP			
Client Choice - Glutes, Hamstrings, Lats				
	3	8-12		60 sec
	3	8-12		60 sec
	3	8-12		60 sec
	3	8-12		60 sec
Cardio, Core, and Cool Down				
Cardio	n/a	n/a	n/a	n/a
Glute Bridge March	3	8-12		60 sec
Hyperexstensions	3	12-15		60 sec
Static Stretching	n/a	n/a		45 seconds

Block 5

(Repeat for 3 weeks, then deload)

Exercise	Sets	Reps	Weight	Rest Period
Mobility and Activation				
IYT Raises Chest Supported	2	6-8		45 sec
Dislocations	2	6-8		45 sec
DB Bench press	2	25		45 sec
Resistance Training				
Bench Press	3	3-5		120 sec
Paused Bench Press	6	3	80% of heaviest bench that day	45 sec
Pec Flys	5	8-10		90 sec
JM Press	4	6-8		
Lifters Choice - Chest, Triceps, Biceps				
	3	8-10		60 sec
	3	8-10		60 sec
	3	8-10		60 sec
	3	8-10		60 sec
Cardio, Core, and Cool Down				
Cardio	n/a	n/a	n/a	n/a
Ab wheel or BB rollout	3	12-15		60sec
Eccentric Decline Situps Tempo (0.0.6)	3	8-12		60sec
Static Stretching	n/a	n/a	n/a	45 sec

Exercise	Sets	Reps	Weight	Rest Period
Mobility and Activation				
Kneeling hip extensions	2	6-8		45 sec
Elevated Touch downs	2	8-12		45 sec
Cossack Squats	2	8-12		45 sec
Resistance Training				
Squats	3	3-5		120 sec
Paused Squats	6	3	80% of heaviest squat that day	45 sec
DB RDL	4	8-12		60 sec
Landmine Rows	5	8-12		90 sec
Lifters Choice - Quads, Calves, Upper Back				
	3	8-10		60 sec
	3	8-10		60 sec
	3	8-10		60 sec
	3	8-10		60 sec
Cardio, Core, and Cool Down				
Cardio	n/a	n/a	n/a	n/a
Hanging Leg Lifts	3	8-12		60 sec
Landmine Oblique twists	3	12-15		60 sec
Static Stretching	n/a	n/a	n/a	45sec

Exercise	Sets	Reps	Weight	Rest Period
Mobility and Activation				
External and Internal Shoulder Rotations	2	12-15		45 sec
DB Reverse Flys	3	8-12		45 sec
Standing DB Overhead press	2	25		45 sec
Resistance Training				
Seated Overhead Press	6	6-8		120 sec
Seated DB Lateral Raises	4	8-12		90 sec
Skullcrushers	5	8-12		90 sec
Swinging Hammer Curls	4	6-8		120 sec
Lifters Choice - Deltoids, triceps, Biceps				
	3	8-10		60 sec
	3	8-10		60 sec
	3	8-10		60 sec
	3	8-10		60 sec
Cardio, Core, and Cool Down				
Cardio	n/a	n/a	n/a	n/a
Crunches - Paused	4	25		
Suitcase Carries - heavy	3	50 ft		60 sec
Static Stretching	n/a	n/a	n/a	45 seconds

Exercise	Sets	Reps	Weight	Rest Period
Mobility and Activation				
Cat Cows	2	6-8		45 sec
Kneeling Kettle Bell Shifts	2	6-8		45 sec
Step ups	3	8-12		45 sec
Resistance Training				
Deadlifts	3	4-6		120 sec
Deadlifts - Speed	6	3	80% of heaviest deadlift that day	90 sec
Incline Chest supported rows	4	6-8		90 sec
Lat Pulldowns - Tempo (0.2.6)	5	8-12		
Client Choice - Glutes, Hamstrings, Lats				
	3	8-10		60 sec
	3	8-10		60 sec
	3	8-10		60 sec
	3	8-10		60 sec
Cardio, Core, and Cool Down				
Cardio	n/a	n/a	n/a	n/a
Superman - Paused	3	12-15		60 sec
Kettlebell Bridge Pullover	3	6-12		60 sec
Static Stretching	n/a	n/a		45 seconds

PART 3

Appendix A
Exercise Selection

The list of exercises is meant to be used as additional work in your resistance training. Listen to your body when performing these exercises. If something feels uncomfortable or is causing pain, stop immediately. If you do not recognize or know n exercise on the list or even in the program, then use google or YouTube. I tried my best to explain the exercises, but I understand many of you may be visual learners and need to see the exercises performed. YouTube can be your best friend in this regard.

Chest	Upper Back	Lats	Quads	Hamstrings
DB Bench	Landmine Row	Lat Pulldown	Leg Exstensions	Hamstring Curls
DB Incline Bench	Machine Row	Lat Pushdown	Goblet Squats	Romanian Deadlifts
DB Decline Bench	Cable Low Rows	Pullover	Heel Elevated Squats	Good Mornings
Machine Chest Press	Shrugs	Pull Up	Hack Squat	Nordic Curls
DB Flys	Seal Row	Chin Up	Sissy Squat	Leg Press
DB Incline Fly	DB Row	Nuetral Grip Pullup	Split Squat	Single Leg Deadlift
Machine Fly	Bent Over Row	Single Arm Pulldown	Lumberjack Squat	Lunges
Cable Flys	Penlay Row	Machine High Row		Glute Ham Raises
Plate Press	T-bar Row			
Pushup				
DB Floor Press				

Glutes	Biceps	Triceps	Deltoids	Calves
Hip Thrusts	EZ Bar Curls	Tricep Rope Pushdown	Lateral Raise	BB Calf Raises
Cable Pullthrough	DB Alternating curls	Tricep Straight bar Pushdown	Front Raise	Smith machine Calf Raises
Cable Kickbacks	Hammer Curls	Close Grip Bench	Rear Delt Fly	Seated DB Calf Raises
Back Exstensions	Cable Curls	Behind the head tricep exstension DB/cable/ez bar	Rear Delt DB Fly	Standing Machine Calf Raises
Hip Abduction	Spider Curls	Rolling Tricep Exstension	Shoulder Press	Seated Machine Calf Raises
Hip Adduction	Inclined Curls	JM Press	Arnold Press	Donkey Calf Raises
Sumo Squat	Superman Curls	Skullcrusher DB or EZ bar	Face Pulls	
Floor Bridge	Preacher Curls	Machine Tricep	Landmine Press	
Donkey Kicks	DB Preacher Curls	Floor Press	IYT Raises	
	Drag Curls		DB Shoulder Press	
	Machine Curls		Cable Rear Delt fly	

Cardio Exercises

This is the section you can just ignore. Nobody likes cardio. But it is good for our bodies. Cardiovascular health is very important for being healthy. Cardio is also great for burning lots of calories. There is a popular misconception that cardio burns fat. This is not true. Cardio burns calories and being in a calorie deficit burns fat. I will give you a few ways to perform your cardio. Keep in mind that these are just ways to do cardio in the gym. You can always go out for a walk or jog, or even a hike in the woods. I include multiple ways to perform cardio on each of these.

The first way is called steady state. Your go for time or distance and attempt to maintain a specific pace with you increase week by week.

Example:

Week 1: Treadmill set to 3 incline at a pace of 3.5 for 20 minutes.

Week 2: Treadmill set to 3.5 incline at a pace of 4 for 20 minutes.

Week 3: Treadmill set to 4 incline at a pace of 4 for 20 minutes.

On week 2 you realize that a pace of 4 is hard enough and any higher and you may not finish, so you keep the same pace but increase the incline. You keep doing this until you hit a point where you cannot keep the pace. Some people may prefer this style of cardio. I personally do not as I get bored easily. I have found that setting my phone up and watching something like a show or YouTube videos makes it easier.

Treadmill	Set speed and try to stay at that speed for a set time. Increase incline to increase difficulty. 20 min is a good start point. Increase as needed.
Elliptical	Same as treadmill. Add sprints. 30/60 or 60/120 depending on the level of difficulty. Sprint as hard as possible for 30 seconds then walk for 60. same with 60/120
Stationary Bicycle	Same as elliptical and treadmill. Can do distance, time, or sprints.
Rower	Choose a distance and row as hard as possible to reach that distance. Can also do timed.
Stair Monster	Again, for time or go for number of stair flights.
Bag Work	Set a timer for 65 seconds. Punch, kick, elbow, knee, headbutt the bag nonstop until the timer is done. Rest for 30 seconds and repeat for 6,8, or 10 rounds.

The second style of cardio is hiit style or High Intensity Interval Training. This type of cardio is designed to have you push as hard as you can for a specific time or number of reps followed by a short rest period. After the short rest period you perform the same exercise again. I personally prefer hiit style cardio as I can put all my energy into the exercise to get through it faster. You can perform hiit style cardio in different ways. One way is sprints. Go as hard as you can for 30 seconds, then rest for 60 seconds. Repeat for 6-10 rounds. Another way is bag work. The last way is to use the spreadsheet included in this appendix and put together your own hiit workout.

The exercises should be performed as followed:

1. Exercise 1 – your choice from column 1 – performed for a set distance.
2. Exercise 2 – Your choice from column 2 - performed for 8-12 reps
3. Exercise 3 - Your choice from column 3 - performed for distance.
4. Exercise 4 - Your choice from column 4 - performed for 12-15 reps

An example hiit workout would be:

1. Sled push down and back equal to 50ft
2. Burpees for 8-12 reps
3. Suicide sprints down and back for 3 reps
4. Russian Twists 12-15 reps

You would perform all 4 exercises without resting between them and then rest for 30-60 seconds. You would then repeat from number 1 again for 3-6 total rounds.

HIIT			
Workout 1 -Distance	Workout 2 - Reps	Workout 3 - Distance	Wokout 4 - Reps
Sled Push	Pushup	Suicide Sprints	Crunches
Sled Pull	Pullup	High Knee	Plank
Sled Explosive Pulls	Dip	Butt Kickers	Hanging leg raises
Farmer Carries	Burpees	Squat to Jump Forward	Leg Raises
Suitcase Carries	Lunges	Bear Crawls	6' Inches
KB Overhead Carries	Jump Squat	Inch worms	Butterfly Kicks
DB Overhead Carries	Jumping Jack	Workout 1 Column	Mountain Climbers
Power Cleans	Step Up		Russian Twists
DB Cleans to Press	Box Jump		Feet in TRX Knees to chest
DB Romanian Deadlift to URR	Jump Rope		Bicycle Crunch
Kettlebell Swings	Jump Lunges		Plank Jacks
Battle Ropes	Side Lunges		Ball Slams
Squat to Ball Throws	Tuck Jumps		Wall Balls

About the Author

Before I found the gym, I was a fat awkward kid. I was introduced to the gym in high school where I quickly fell in love with the feel of iron in my hands. The gym gave me confidence and helped mold me into who I am today. After High School I enlisted in the Army where I learned to step out of my comfort zone, push myself to the limit, and chase after goals I am passionate about. I spent 3 years serving in the Infantry before being Honorably Discharged. I attended the Physical Therapy Assistance program at Keiser University and obtained my NASM personal trainer certificate through online courses. I am always researching and educating myself on all things fitness. I met the love of my life, got married, and began growing our family. They have always been supportive of me, my goals, and are always cheering the loudest at all my competitions. I wouldn't be the man I am today without them.

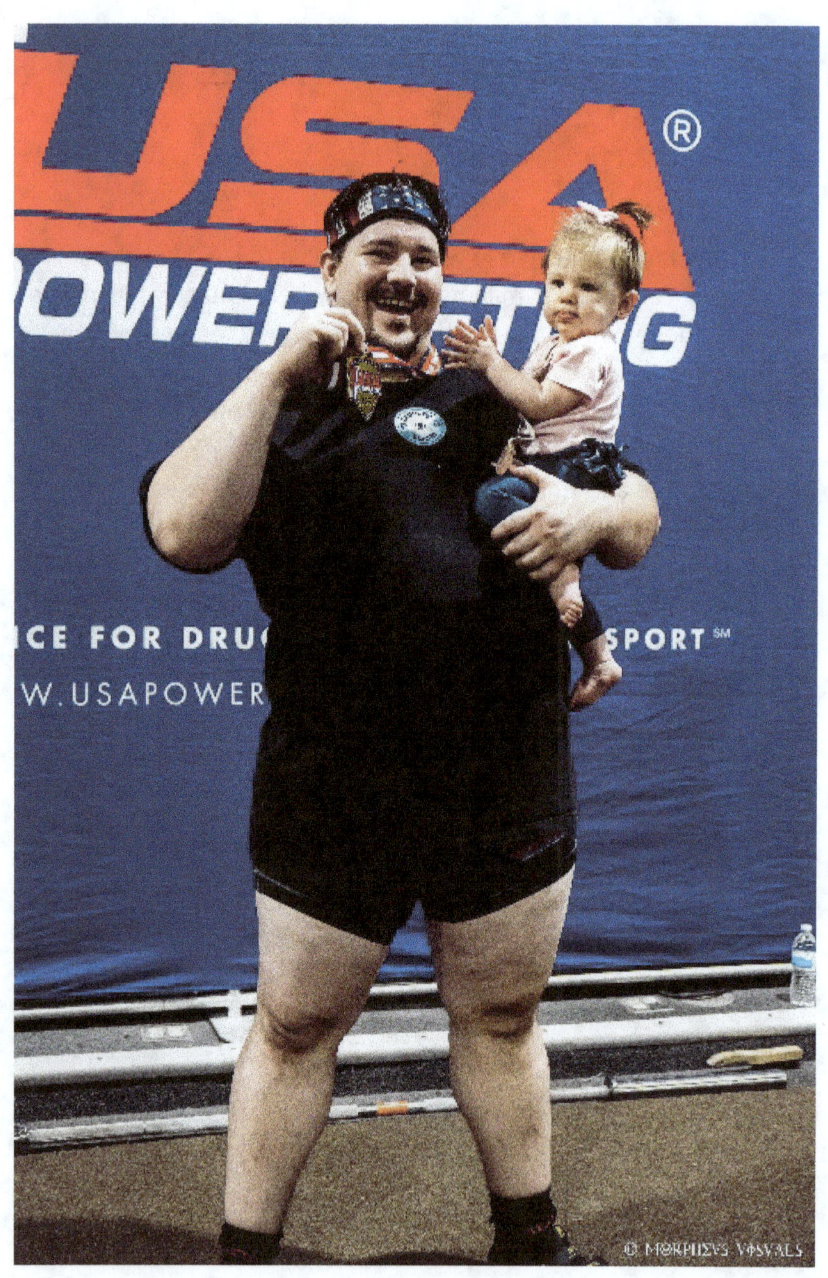

USA
POWERLIFTING
ICE FOR DRUG   SPORT℠
W.USAPOWER
© MORPHEUS VISUALS

www.ingramcontent.com/pod-product-compliance
Lightning Source LLC
Chambersburg PA
CBHW070856260726
48661CB00004B/1446